School-Based Crisis Intervention

THE GUILFORD PRACTICAL INTERVENTION IN THE SCHOOLS SERIES

Kenneth W. Merrell, Series Editor

Books in this series address the complex academic, behavioral, and social–emotional needs of children and youth at risk. School-based practitioners are provided with practical, research-based, and readily applicable tools to support students and team successfully with teachers, families, and administrators. Each volume is designed to be used directly and frequently in planning and delivering clinical services. Features include a convenient format to facilitate photocopying, step-by-step instructions for assessment and intervention, and helpful, timesaving reproducibles.

Helping Students Overcome Depression and Anxiety: A Practical Guide
Kenneth W. Merrell

Emotional and Behavioral Problems of Young Children: Effective Interventions in the Preschool and Kindergarten Years
Gretchen A. Gimpel and Melissa L. Holland

Conducting School-Based Functional Behavioral Assessments:
A Practitioner's Guide
T. Steuart Watson and Mark W. Steege

Executive Skills in Children and Adolescents: A Practical Guide to Assessment and Intervention
Peg Dawson and Richard Guare

Responding to Problem Behavior in Schools: The Behavior Education Program
Deanne A. Crone, Robert H. Horner, and Leanne S. Hawken

Resilient Classrooms: Creating Healthy Environments for Learning
Beth Doll, Steven Zucker, and Katherine Brehm

Helping Schoolchildren with Chronic Health Conditions:
A Practical Guide
Daniel L. Clay

Interventions for Reading Problems: Designing and Evaluating Effective Strategies
Edward J. Daly III, Sandra Chafouleas, and Christopher H. Skinner

Safe and Healthy Schools: Practical Prevention Strategies
Jeffrey R. Sprague and Hill M. Walker

School-Based Crisis Intervention: Preparing All Personnel to Assist
Melissa Allen Heath and Dawn Sheen

School-Based Crisis Intervention

Preparing All Personnel to Assist

MELISSA ALLEN HEATH
DAWN SHEEN

THE GUILFORD PRESS
New York   London

© 2005 The Guilford Press
A Division of Guilford Publications, Inc.
72 Spring Street, New York, NY 10012
www.guilford.com

Printed in Canada

This book is printed on acid-free paper.

Last digit is print number: 9   8   7   6   5   4   3   2   1

Library of Congress Cataloging-in-Publication Data

Heath, Melissa Allen.
   School-based crisis intervention : preparing all personnel to assist / Melissa Allen Heath,
Dawn Sheen.
      p. cm. — (The Guilford practical intervention in the schools series)
   ISBN 1-59385-151-0
   1. School crisis management.   2. Crisis intervention (Mental health services)   I. Sheen,
Dawn.   II. Title.   III. Series.
   LB2866.5.H43 2005
   363.11'9371—dc22
                                                                            2004030977

About the Authors

Melissa Allen Heath, PhD, is an assistant professor in the Department of Counseling Psychology and Special Education at Brigham Young University. Her primary research interest is crisis prevention and intervention in the school setting. She is a licensed psychologist and a nationally and state-certified school psychologist. In addition to serving on school, district, and community crisis teams, she also received crisis training through the Red Cross Community Emergency Response Team (CERT) programs. Over the past 10 years, she has worked with schools and communities in developing basic training materials for crisis intervention.

Dawn Sheen is currently a master's student in school psychology at Brigham Young University. Prior to graduate school, she was a middle school teacher specializing in multicultural awareness and French and Spanish language instruction. Her previous experience with crisis intervention includes managing a women's shelter for those affected by domestic violence and assisting with a community rape crisis hotline. Recognizing the need for student involvement with disaster preparedness, she sponsored an after-school "Masters of Disaster" class taught in conjunction with the Red Cross. Her research interests include crisis prevention and intervention as well as multicultural issues in school settings.

Preface

STATEMENT OF PURPOSE

During stressful times, students look to and rely on adults for direction, stability, and caring reassurance (Johnson, 1998). This support is needed not only for times of extreme crisis, but more importantly for the daily challenges of maintaining a safe and nurturing environment conducive to learning. Providing this support in the form of emotional first aid is an often overlooked aspect of working with children and youth in school settings.

This book is designed to assist *all* adults, including mental health professionals, teachers, and staff, in providing emotional first aid for students. We present basic intervention skills—how to react, what to say, and what to do—as well as information, strategies, and resources on a wide variety of crisis intervention topics. We also offer ideas for staff inservice training with the goal of preparing *all* adults to better meet the emotional needs of students.

SCHOOL-BASED MENTAL HEALTH SERVICES

Over the past decade, the challenge of meeting children's mental health needs, including crisis intervention, has increasingly become the responsibility of school-based mental health professionals (Brock, Sandoval, & Lewis, 2001; Johnson, 2000). In order to increase the availability of services for children, professionals are encouraged to meet the needs of children and families "where they are" (U.S. Department of Health and Human Services, 2000).

The pressure to provide emotional support within public schools comes from a variety of political, societal, and individual family factors. First and foremost, school is where children and adolescents receive the bulk of mental health care: 75% of mental health services for children and adolescents is provided in the context of public schools (Burns & Hoagwood, 2002). Because most youth under the age of 18 spend approximately one third of their waking hours in school, providing crisis intervention services within the framework of the school is natural and appropriate. Although it might seem that school mental health professionals have the benefit of being able to link into the school's convenient and natural support system automatically, the word *automatically* oversimplifies the difficulties of providing crisis intervention to large numbers of children in the wake of traumatic events. Even more pressing, limited professional resources and mental health services are stretched, on a daily basis, to adequately support students faced with personal difficulties.

Students' problems, particularly the more visible "acting-out" behaviors such as aggression and hyperactivity, are apparent to teachers. Teachers are on the front line of red-flagging student problems, both behavioral and emotional. Teachers and staff depend on the assistance of professionals in defining, implementing, and monitoring interventions. In addition to helping teachers meet the academic needs of students, mental health services in the school have become a resource for families and communities. When families and teachers understand the emotional issues underlying students' behavioral problems, they are more likely to assist in implementing appropriate interventions to strengthen both academic performance and healthy social adjustment.

Various factors impact the need for children's mental health services. The National Institute of Child Health and Human Development (2003) provided the following information in a publication titled *America's Children: Key National Indicators of Well-Being, 2003*. Almost 16% of children in the United States live in poverty; 36% in homes that are inadequate, crowded, or unsafe; and 18% with insufficient financial resources for adequate nutrition. Almost 6% of children and adolescents have no access to health care; 28% live in single-parent homes; 4% live in "no-parent" homes; and almost 25% of children under the age of 14 have no parental or adult supervision when they come home from school. Considering another indicator of compromised emotional and social well-being, almost 20% of all serious crimes are committed by adolescents.

These facts are alarming, leaving one feeling overwhelmed with the challenge of meeting children's needs. Schools, in particular, are burdened with the effects of so many negative forces in today's society. In addition to teaching academics, schools have increasingly taken on other responsibilities, such as preschool services, full-day kindergarten, after-school programs, and feeding children breakfast, lunch, and snacks. Still, faced with all of these challenges, those in the teaching and helping professions continue to pose these questions: "How can we help? How can we make a difference?"

Because of the vast number of children in comparison to the limited number of mental health professionals in the schools—47 million students to only 90,000 school counselors and 30,000 school psychologists—resources are stretched to meet the vast and varied mental health needs of students. This means that in schools nationwide the ratio is approximately 400 students per mental health professional.

Realizing that the emotional needs of students exceed available professional resources, we propose that all adults in the school, with minimal preparation, can assist in providing basic emotional support to students. This idea of training all adults in schools to provide basic emotional first aid is similar to the Red Cross strategy of training laypeople to care for immediate medical needs in emergency situations. Although laypeople are not trained to perform complex medical procedures, and are not expected to act outside of their limited area of training, they can and do perform life-saving first-aid procedures. Likewise, adults in schools, if properly trained, can provide basic emotional support to students experiencing stress and trauma.

The unique feature of this book that sets it apart from other school crisis publications is the inclusion of information and training guidelines for the total school staff: teachers, teaching assistants, secretarial staff, bus drivers, and custodial staff. Preparing all adults who interact with students on a daily basis will provide a stronger and more supportive school environment, fostering resilience and buffering the negative impact of stressful situations (APA Task Force on Resilience, 2002).

GOALS AND OBJECTIVES

Most books dealing with crisis intervention have focused on meeting the needs of adults, with minimal content regarding children and even less content related to schools. However, over the past decade there has been a growing interest in school crisis intervention, evidenced by a marked increase in publications dealing with this topic. Even so, crisis intervention books and training programs currently on the market, although useful, fall short of reaching the broad audience of *all adults* in the school system. Academic books and training materials speak the language of professionals and often lack the critical and practical "how-to" information for effectively implementing schoolwide crisis prevention and intervention programs. Additionally, most training materials for crisis intervention focus on large-scale or high-profile situations rather than on more commonly occurring situations.

The objective of this book is to prepare *all* school staff to provide emotional first aid—not just for those in acute crisis, but also for those in need of a helping hand or a listening ear. A broader base of emotional support will bolster students' transition through difficult times.

Information in this book is geared toward providing all staff with a basic understanding of crisis intervention. Topics include fostering a supportive, inclusive, and positive school climate; providing effective crisis intervention for students from diverse backgrounds; using basic communication skills in providing emotional support; communicating with community mental health professionals, parents, and the media; utilizing children's literature to strengthen students' coping skills; and strategies for avoiding burnout.

A portion of the book is devoted to inservice training activities that focus on what to say, what to do, and when to refer students to mental health professionals. More specifically, the information provided is aimed at training staff to listen carefully to and communicate with students, parents/guardians, teachers, and other professionals concerning students' emotional needs, particularly during difficult and traumatic times.

Chapter 5, "Assisting Students with Specific Problems," goes into more detail about specific topics, including depression, anxiety, chronic illness, difficulties in making and keeping friends, divorce, parent problems, abuse, financial difficulties, suicide, and grief and loss issues. Additionally, Chapter 5 provides ideas and resources for classroom activities that can be conducted easily with minimal advance preparation. Suggested stories and activities target common difficulties children face and are clearly outlined for fast and easy delivery. These resources assist staff and teachers in strengthening students' coping skills and bolstering a sense of community and caring support.

PROPOSED AUDIENCE

This book has a schoolwide focus; our intention is to provide teaching materials and basic crisis intervention strategies for use by school psychologists, counselors, social workers, teachers, and support staff. The emphasis on training all staff for crisis intervention makes this book a practical guide for university training programs that prepare school-based professionals, including educational administration, teacher education, school psychology, social work, and school counseling. School-based professionals will find the handouts and overheads helpful in planning staff development and inservice training.

Contents

List of Worksheets, Handouts, Overheads, Tables, and Figure   xv

1. **Introduction to Crisis Intervention**   1
   MELISSA ALLEN HEATH, DAWN SHEEN, ELLIE L. YOUNG, AND BART LYMAN
   Defining a Crisis and Levels of Intervention   2
   Prevention: Fostering a Supportive, Inclusive, and Positive School Climate   4
   Targeting Bullying and Harassment   6
   Suggested Learning Activities for Teacher and Staff Training   8
   Student Response to Emotional Stress and Trauma   10

2. **Responding to a Crisis**   23
   MELISSA ALLEN HEATH, DAWN SHEEN, NEIL ANNANDALE, AND BART LYMAN
   What Is a School Crisis Plan?   24
   Common Problems with Crisis Plans   25
   What Is a Crisis Team?   26
   Control and Organization during a School Crisis   27
   Classroom Emergency Kits   27
   Roles and Responsibilities of Each Adult   28
   A Crisis Plan in Action   29
   Effective Crisis Intervention for Students from Diverse Backgrounds   31
       The Stockton Schoolyard Shootings   32
   Current School Demographics   32
       Ethnic Diversity   32
       Linguistic Diversity   33
   Matching Services to Multicultural Needs   33
   Planning and Conducting a Multicultural Needs Assessment   34

3. **Communication: How to Listen, What to Say, and How to React**   44
   MELISSA ALLEN HEATH AND ANNETTE JEROME
   Referring to a Professional   45
   Strengthening Communication Skills   45
   Listening to Students in Crisis: Basic Listening Skills   46
       Position   46
       Body Language   47
       Speech   48
       Action Plan   48
       Follow-Up   48
   Teaching Listening Skills   49
       Video Clip: City Slickers   50

Video Clip: A Christmas Story 51
Video Clip: As Good as It Gets 53
Summary of Good Listening Skills 53
Communicating with Community Mental Health Professionals 54
Reporting Suspected Abuse 55
Communicating with Parents 55
Communicating with the Media 56

4. Children's Literature: A Resource to Assist with Crisis Intervention　　64
DAWN SHEEN, MELISSA ALLEN HEATH, NATHAN JONES, EMILY HEATON,
AND APRIL GSTETTENBAUER

What Is Bibliotherapy? 65
Stages of Bibliotherapy 66
Literature Selection 66
Teaching Process 67
Signs of Distress 68
Summary 69
Additional Materials 69

5. Assisting Students with Specific Problems　　77
DAWN SHEEN, MELISSA ALLEN HEATH, JOLENE CAMPBELL, CHRISANDRA MELVILLE,
AND BART LYMAN

Depression 78
Anxiety 79
Chronic Illness 79
Difficulties Making and Keeping Friends 80
Divorce 80
Problems at Home 81
Abuse 81
Suicide 82
Death and Grieving 83
Staff Training Handouts 84
Handout and Overhead Topics 84
Bibliotherapy Activities 85
Suggested Books 85
Classroom Activities 85
Activities for Mental Health Professionals 89
Additional Activities 90
Activities Related to Feelings 91
Getting to Know You Activities 97
Teamwork Activities 98
Communication Activities 99
Problem-Solving Activities 100
Self-Image Activity 101

6. Preparing Noninstructional Personnel and Bus Drivers to Assist　　142
with Crisis Prevention and Intervention
MELISSA ALLEN HEATH AND ELLIE L. YOUNG

Preparing Bus Drivers to Assist 143
Preparing Custodial Staff and Cafeteria Workers to Assist 144
Conducting Staff Training 144
Crisis Intervention Topics for Noninstructional Staff 146
Inventory of Staff Skills 147
Guidelines for Involving Staff in Crisis Intervention 147

7. Avoiding Burnout: Taking Care of Yourself 150

MELISSA ALLEN HEATH AND BART LYMAN

What Is Burnout? 151
Factors That Increase Stress 152
Symptoms of Burnout 153
Keeping Yourself Emotionally Healthy 153
  Evaluate Your Strengths and Weaknesses 154
  Share and Delegate Responsibilities 154
  Maintain Appropriate Boundaries 155
  Develop Support Networks 155
  Stress-Reducing Activities 156
  Staff and Teacher Training Activity 157
Conclusion 157

APPENDIX A. Free Crisis Intervention Resources from the Substance Abuse 161
and Mental Health Services Administration

APPENDIX B. Additional Books for Bibliotherapy 164

References 167

Index 171

List of Worksheets, Handouts, Overheads, Tables, and Figure

WORKSHEETS

WORKSHEET 1.1. Behavior Problems: What, Where, and How Often   14

WORKSHEET 3.1. Listening Skills (Part 1)   58

WORKSHEET 3.2. Listening Skills (Part 2)   59

WORKSHEET 3.3. Emergency Contact Log   60

WORKSHEET 4.1. Bibliotherapy Summary   73

WORKSHEET 4.2. Expressing Our Feelings   74

WORKSHEET 5.1. Thoughts Connect with Feelings (Ages 8 and Older)   104

WORKSHEET 5.2. We Aren't "Bugged"! (Teacher Copy)   105

WORKSHEET 5.3. We Aren't "Bugged"!   106

WORKSHEET 5.4. Divorce Worksheet (Ages 8–12)   107

WORKSHEET 5.5. Feelings about Divorce (Ages 6–12)   108

WORKSHEET 5.6. Masks (Ages 5–11)   109

WORKSHEET 5.7. Masks (Ages 12–18)   110

WORKSHEET 5.8. Problem-Solving Steps (Ages 8 and Older)   111

WORKSHEET 6.1. Crisis Intervention   149

HANDOUTS

HANDOUT 1.1. Bullying   15

HANDOUT 1.2. Decreasing Bullying   16

HANDOUT 1.3. Violence   17

HANDOUT 2.1. Diversity in Our Schools   40

HANDOUT 2.2. Questions about Your School Crisis Plan   41

HANDOUT 2.3. Role Playing Crisis Scenarios   42

HANDOUT 3.1. Listening to Students in Crisis: Basic Listening Skills   61

HANDOUT 4.1. Evaluating Literature for Bibliotherapy   75

HANDOUT 5.1. Topic: Depression   112

HANDOUT 5.2. Topic: Chronic and Serious Illness   113

HANDOUT 5.3. Topic: Difficulties Making and Keeping Friends   114

HANDOUT 5.4. Topic: Divorce   115

HANDOUT 5.5. Topic: Abuse   116

HANDOUT 5.6. Topic: Abuse   117

HANDOUT 5.7. Topic: Suicide   118

HANDOUT 5.8. Topic: Death and Grief   119

HANDOUT 5.9. Grief   120

HANDOUT 5.10. Sea Glass   121

HANDOUT 7.1. Preventing Burnout: Keeping Yourself Emotionally Healthy   159

OVERHEADS

OVERHEAD 1.1. Bullying   18

OVERHEAD 1.2. Decrease Bullying by Increasing A.W.A.R.E.N.E.S.S.   19

OVERHEAD 1.3. Stop Sexual Harassment   20

OVERHEAD 1.4. Violence Prevention = Positive School Climate   21

OVERHEAD 2.1. Crisis Response Skills   43

OVERHEAD 3.1. Fundamentals of Good Listening   62

OVERHEAD 3.2. Stay Calm   63

OVERHEAD 4.1. Purposes and Stages of Bibliotherapy   76

OVERHEAD 5.1. Abuse: What You Can Do   122

OVERHEAD 5.2. Abuse   123

OVERHEAD 5.3. Signs of Abuse   124

OVERHEAD 5.4. Crying For Help   125

OVERHEAD 5.5. If a Student Is Thinking about Suicide   126

OVERHEAD 5.6. The Mourning Process   127

OVERHEAD 5.7. Defining Group Rules   128

OVERHEAD 5.8. Problem-Solving Steps   129

OVERHEAD 5.9. Anxiety   130

TABLES

TABLE 1.1. Reactions to Stress and Trauma   11

TABLE 3.1. Cueing Video Clips for Listening Skills   50

TABLE 7.1. Symptoms of Burnout   153

FIGURE

FIGURE 5.1. Suggested activities, topics addressed, and conditions/problems   86
to which they apply.

1

Introduction to Crisis Intervention

MELISSA ALLEN HEATH, DAWN SHEEN, ELLIE L. YOUNG, *and* BART LYMAN

CRISIS INTERVENTION: A BRIEF OVERVIEW

Receiving immediate emotional first aid is crucial in assisting students and staff to cope and adjust. The stabilizing effect of immediate care and support cannot be underestimated. Eric Lindemann (1944, 1979) brought this point to the public's attention following the 1942 Cocoanut Grove nightclub fire in Boston. Families were celebrating after the Harvard–Yale football game when the overcrowded nightclub caught fire. Flames quickly consumed the building, killing almost 500 people. Physicians, emergency medical technicians, nurses, mental health professionals, clergy, and community volunteers assisted with the emergency and subsequently with survivors and families of the deceased. Lindemann noted that this immediate support facilitated the survivors' grieving process and assisted them in adjusting to their loss and ultimately adapting to their new life. Those receiving immediate intervention appeared to suffer less maladjustment later in life.

Another example of crisis intervention, this time specifically related to children, occurred in 1976 when three masked men hijacked a busload of 26 children in Chowchilla, California. Threatening the driver and children with a gun, the hijackers drove the bus to a remote location in the desert. Here the children were transferred to a trailer in a ravine and covered over with dirt. The children remained in the buried vehicle until they were rescued 27 hours after being abducted. After returning to their families, everyone's immediate focus was on the physical condition of the children. Much to the parents' relief, the

Ellie L. Young, PhD, Assistant Professor, Department of Counseling Psychology Special Education, Brigham Young University, Provo, Utah.

Bart Lyman, BS, graduate student in School Psychology Program, Brigham Young University, Provo, Utah.

children appeared to be physically unharmed. Everyone wanted to put the incident behind them. They wanted to go on with life as it had been before the abduction. None of the children received crisis intervention counseling. Four years later, Terr (1983) followed up on these same children and reported that most of them continued to experience emotional difficulties related to the traumatic incident, particularly high levels of anxiety and recurring nightmares. Terr explained that the children's unresolved trauma was most likely related to the absence of immediate crisis intervention following their rescue. Her work emphasized the need to focus on more than just physical well-being. She stressed the importance of focusing on emotional well-being in order to prevent long-term emotional difficulties.

In contrasting the outcomes of crisis intervention for the Cocoanut Grove fire and the Chowchilla school bus incident, the difference in victims' recovery appeared to be contingent on receiving immediate emotional first aid rendered by volunteers and professionals. Based on Lindemann's (1979) observations, it could be concluded that long-term effects of the Cocoanut Grove tragedy were greatly reduced because immediate emotional support was provided.

DEFINING A CRISIS AND LEVELS OF INTERVENTION

What is a crisis? A *crisis* is an event or circumstance that occurs often without warning and initially poses an overwhelming threat to an individual or group. Dealing with the immediate and ensuing difficulties that arise from a crisis requires greater resources than are readily available to the individual or group. Simply stated, the demands exceed the resources.

In a school setting, crises expose students and staff to threat, loss, and traumatic stimuli, creating chaos and threatening safety, security, and stability. A crisis may affect large numbers of students and staff or may be confined to a small group or even an individual. Schoolwide trauma may include suicides, accidents, incidents of violence, school shootings, bomb threats, gang activity, natural disasters, medical emergencies, or community or national disasters. Crises affecting an individual or small group may include divorce, grief, loss, bullying, drug abuse, abuse (emotional, physical, or sexual), and chronic or acute illness.

A crisis occurring during school hours upsets order and the normal routine of students. Panic and confusion escalate, overwhelming the helping capacity of even trained professionals. Given the large number of children and families served, it is unrealistic to expect one school social worker, school counselor, or school psychologist to provide individualized "psychological first aid" to hundreds, even thousands, of students and adults during a crisis.

In planning for crisis intervention, it is important to consider the number of individuals who may be affected by different tragedies. In preparation for meeting demands of a school crisis, basic training must be offered to all adults in the school. Brock et al. (2001) state that a crisis plan "is useless without personnel capable of conducting crisis interventions" (p. 52). As administrators and mental health professionals formulate crisis plans and consider training needs, it is imperative to plan and prepare for three levels of crisis intervention: primary, secondary, and tertiary (Caplan, 1964).

Primary intervention includes preventive efforts that (1) lessen the likelihood of a crisis; (2) reduce the extent and magnitude of trauma in the event a crisis occurs; and (3) assist in inoculating students against stressors, strengthening their coping skills, and fortifying them against negative forces. In an attempt to improve school climate and safety, schoolwide programs may target unacceptable behavior such as bullying, sexual harassment, violence, and drugs. Other programs may take on a positive approach, targeting prosocial behavior such as improving student leadership, character development, citizenship, community service, mentoring, peer mediation, and conflict resolution skills. Most of these programs foster personal responsibility and focus on strengthening a caring, inclusive school climate.

Although prevention should be a major focus of all school crisis plans, most crisis plans deal primarily with *secondary intervention*: planning for the acute phase of crisis. Crisis plans outline strategies and organize energy and resources to help with immediate demands during a crisis. Frequently these plans outline services provided by crisis teams, comprised of school mental health professionals and other staff within the individual school or school district. Additionally, counselors and professionals from the community may participate as members of a school's crisis team.

Although counselors and professionals outside the school system may assist with crisis intervention, particularly during large-scale incidents, administrators typically voice concerns about depending on "outsiders" (Johnson, 2000; Poland, Pitcher, & Lazarus, 1999). Those working in school systems note that outside professionals have difficulty interfacing with schools, and although their desires are well intentioned, outside services may be perceived as intrusive, overreactive, and misaligned with a particular school's power structure and organization. Unless there is a strong ongoing relationship between the school and the outside professionals and unless services are properly coordinated, outside assistance adds to confusion, increases the stress of an already difficult situation, and ultimately fosters feelings of frustration, helplessness, and inadequacy in the school's staff (Weinberg, 1989). Additionally, students' feelings of trust and security may be jeopardized when unfamiliar professionals assist in providing emotional support.

Although dramatic events covered by the media such as school shootings, bomb threats, and natural disasters garner the bulk of public attention, providing secondary intervention for a wide variety and level of emotional needs is of paramount importance. In addition to major schoolwide crises, students are also challenged by individual crises such as family problems, illness, divorce, death of a pet, bullying, and so on. Although these crises may seem almost insignificant when compared to the mass devastation of a school shooting, they comprise the bulk of incidents occurring in schools. On a daily basis, teachers and staff assist students in need of emotional support.

After meeting the immediate needs of a crisis situation, the initial shock and overwhelming demands taper off in urgency. However, some students may need ongoing assistance. *Tertiary intervention* targets lingering chronic emotional needs. An extreme example of this level of intervention would be the provision of follow-up efforts a few weeks after a school shooting. Tertiary intervention is extended to those directly affected by tragedy as well as to those peripheral to the event but in need of stabilizing support. Supportive counseling extends beyond the initial tragedy and focuses on coping, adjusting, and healing. Ongoing support assists students in making sense of loss and moving beyond the initial shock of the tragedy.

In addition to ongoing supportive counseling, teachers and staff who work with students on a daily basis also play an important role in providing long-term emotional support. Students' emotional needs cannot be ignored. Understanding and responding to the ongoing needs of students following a crisis are essential in tailoring instruction to maximize learning.

PREVENTION: FOSTERING A SUPPORTIVE, INCLUSIVE, AND POSITIVE SCHOOL CLIMATE

Rather than putting most of their energy into planning for a major disaster, school personnel must invest more energy into preventing crises. Prevention works best if the entire school is involved. Groundwork for prevention must include the basic and underlying principles of developing a warm, inclusive environment that is nurtured by adults who model a caring attitude. Caring can be demonstrated in a variety of ways: One simple way is to greet students each morning. One middle school principal from Texas has a "principal's moment" every morning. Over the intercom, he energetically welcomes everyone to a new day of learning. After greeting the student body, he reads a brief story, fueling the start of a good day. His stories are inspirational, similar to those in the popular series *Chicken Soup for the Soul*. Each story takes about 1 minute for the principal to read and is focused on motivating students to develop strong character and life skills. His enthusiasm and genuine concern for students and staff permeate the school.

As you enter a school, you immediately sense a school's "personality," the principal's leadership, and the character of students and staff. A school's personality goes much deeper than the building's physical appearance. For instance, when the principal and staff greet students and visitors as they enter the building, there is an "unrushed feeling." Taking time to learn students' names and making personal greetings greatly contribute to a positive school climate, which strengthens school unity and student support and provides a comfortable and secure foundation for student learning. Additionally, a positive school climate provides an "umbrella" of order and structure that buffers the effects of negative outside influences. School climate is affected by multiple variables, ranging from external factors such as physical accommodations to the attitudes and internal values of staff and students. The ideal school climate of respect and appreciation for individual differences creates a comfortable atmosphere of acceptance and inclusion.

Suggestions for increasing schoolwide community support include displaying student academic work, decorating halls with student art, visibly celebrating accomplishments, posting banners related to school values and goals, announcing school and community events on bulletin boards, and spotlighting teachers' and students' interests and activities.

Clearly stated, defined, and enforced policies are crucial to the safety and organization of schools. However, a positive school climate also includes a gentler side of concern and care for the individual within the context of the larger group. Although adults in the school are in leadership positions of power and control, school leadership should not be dictatorial. Effective leadership must support collaboration among administrators, teachers, staff, students, and parents. A sense of community, inclusion, and shared responsibility for the welfare of the school, as well as for the individual, supports a positive school climate.

Many benefits accrue to schools that implement strategies to increase positive school climate. Teachers report a higher level of job satisfaction and a reduction in student behavior problems (Guin, 2004). Recent research also suggests that students experience greater positive regard for themselves and others when their school fosters a positive school climate (Ross & Lowther, 2003). Additionally, students report an increased sense of belonging and a positive attitude toward peers, teachers, and administrators. Students who feel connected to their school are less likely to drop out or become involved in delinquent activities.

Practically speaking, a positive school climate can be nurtured in a variety of ways. In addition to learning student names, personalizing hellos, and smiling as students enter the building or classroom, daily demonstration of underlying care and concern for students might include:

- Schoolwide prevention programs targeting problems such as bullying or sexual harassment.
- Schoolwide curriculum and developmental guidance activities promoting respect for diversity and individual differences.
- Student involvement in defining and refining schoolwide and classroom policies.
- Recognition of student, teacher, and staff birthdays.
- Celebration of student success, spotlighting good citizenship, academic achievement, attendance awards, acts of service, and student progress.
- Posters congratulating schoolwide achievements.
- Displays of student work in classrooms, hallways, and cafeteria.
- Shared responsibility for cleaning common areas and classrooms.
- Positive home notes highlighting student accomplishment and appropriate behavior.
- Classroom service projects, offering students opportunities to improve their school and community.
- Planned activities responding to incidents of community, school, or personal loss.

Creating a positive school climate is a group effort, not something one administrator accomplishes independently. Brainstorming and implementing creative ideas tailored to the unique characteristics of the school are critical in fine-tuning a positive school climate. Most importantly, the strategic planning must be followed by action and accountability.

After implementing a plan to improve school climate, monitoring and evaluating efforts may include counting discipline referrals and incidents of fighting, tracking teacher and staff turnover rates, and so on. Additional feedback regarding school climate could be gathered from parents, students, teachers, or staff informally or from surveys soliciting feedback. Other data collection may include monitoring student academic achievement, tardies, dropout rates, homework completion, and involvement with the Parent Teacher Association.

On an individual basis, progress of specific students or groups may be monitored by the school psychologist or school counselor. Analyzing data from formal or informal behavior checklists provides information about student progress over time. For students identified as having special education needs, improvement can be monitored using behavioral goals specified in their individual education plans or behavior improvement plans.

TARGETING BULLYING AND HARASSMENT

Strategically directing more effort into developing a nurturing and caring environment prepares the school to meet critical needs of students and families more effectively. It is important for all adults and students to focus on promoting a positive school climate. A school should "feel good" to students and staff. A schoolwide program to improve school climate may include prevention efforts that target specific behaviors such as bullying and harassment.

Bullying is a form of aggression in which one or more students physically, psychologically, or sexually harass another student repeatedly over time. In this interpersonal context an imbalance of power is perceived whereby the bully is seen as stronger, larger, or older than the targeted individual. Typically incidents of bullying and harassment are unprovoked. Bullies pick on those they believe cannot or will not retaliate.

Bullying and sexual harassment occur frequently in schools. The number of students who report being the target of harassing behaviors ranges from 15% (Olweus, 1993) to 80% (American Association of University Women, 2001). Although estimated frequency of incidents varies depending on the severity of the behavior and how it is defined, harassment of any degree detracts from a positive learning environment.

Some students may be more susceptible to harassment (Kupersmidt & Dodge, 2004; Olweus, 1993). There are two types of targets: passive and provocative. The passive target is described as lonely, without friends, physically weaker, and possibly overprotected by adults. The provocative target is hot-tempered, anxious, high strung, reactive, and has a history of failed attempts to retaliate against the aggressor. It is also important to note that almost 75% of those who have been the target of harassment or bullying go on to harass and bully others. In elementary school the younger children are more likely to be targeted by older children. However, in middle school, students are more likely to bully same-age peers.

There are gender differences in bullying behaviors (Olweus, 1993). In comparison to females, males are three to four times more likely to physically assault their target. Sixty-five percent of bullying is perpetrated by males. Almost 80% of victimized males were bullied by males. In other words, males bully other males. However, it is important not to stereotype bullies.

Gender differences in harassing behaviors have recently been challenged. Current research suggests an increase in females resorting to physical aggression as a method of harassing others (Putallaz & Bierman, 2004). However, although females may physically assault and brutalize others, in general, they are not as likely as males to use physical tactics in bullying. They tend to use "relational aggression" that consists of teasing, ridiculing, excluding others from social groups, starting rumors to embarrass others, and ignoring or treating others as outcasts. Males may also resort to relational aggression when trying to influence or sway peers' opinions or participation in delinquent activities.

Although the frequency of bullying decreases as students reach middle school, sexual harassment increases during middle school years (Yoon, Barton, & Taíariol, 2004). In fact, sexual harassment occurs so commonly in schools, all students, regardless of age or gender, are exposed to the behavior, either personally experiencing sexual harassment or observing the behavior in others.

Broadly defined, sexual harassment is a subcategory of bullying. Sexual harassment may be described as unwanted and unwelcome sexual behaviors or comments considered uncomfortable and offensive by the target. Perpetrators seek to control and embarrass targeted individuals. Examples of sexual harassment include behaviors such as inappropriate touching, groping, swatting the buttocks, pinching, and brushing up against someone in a sexually provocative manner. Other expressions of sexual harassment include sexual comments; name calling (e.g., gay, lesbian, fag); sexual gestures; drawings of sexual graffiti on bathroom walls; sexually oriented jokes, stories, or rumors; display of pornographic pictures; and sexual bribes.

Results of a national survey conducted by the American Association of University Women (2001) indicated that almost equal numbers of boys and girls reported being sexually harassed; however, boys and girls report different types of sexual harassment. Girls report experiencing more physical sexual harassment (inappropriate touching, groping, bra snapping, etc.) as well as more incidents of sexual harassment perpetrated by adults.

Most harassment reported by students occurs in places where adults are present but not closely monitoring student behavior, such as the cafeteria, hallways, and on the school grounds before and after school. Students who are the target of harassment report feeling vulnerable and unsafe. However, feelings of embarrassment make it difficult for them to report incidents to teachers or parents. Males may have a particularly difficult time reporting incidents of sexual harassment perpetrated by females. It is almost as if our culture expects males to enjoy this type of attention. Even when students report harassment, adults may downplay the incident, telling students that the perpetrator was "just joking" or "no harm was meant." In fact, sexual comments and harassing behaviors are so common in middle school that many teachers consider it to be a normal part of growing up.

Because those who bully and sexually harass others often target individuals who are weaker and more vulnerable, students with disabilities are often prime targets. Additionally, students may harass less powerful adults in the school, such as janitors, bus drivers, cafeteria workers, and teaching assistants.

School staff must send a very strong message: *Bullying and harassment will not be tolerated*. Practical suggestions for decreasing bullying and harassment include the following:

- Monitor and assess bullying/harassing behaviors in order to determine seriousness of the problem.
- Actively involve personnel from the top (administration) down. Incorporate anti-bullying/harassment rules into the student code of conduct. Clearly spell out behaviors that will not be tolerated and demonstrate zero tolerance for bullying and harassment.
- Incorporate building-wide interventions. All staff and teachers need training in how to model appropriate behavior and attitude toward bullies and victims. More specifically, they need training in how to react and respond to bullying; they must not ignore students' inappropriate behaviors.
- Choose popular teachers and student leaders to spotlight prosocial behavior and how to react to bullying.
- Desseminate facts about bullying and harassment.
- Provide separate counseling services for perpetrators and targets; provide social skills training for perpetrators and assertiveness training for targets.
- Involve parents in prevention and intervention; however, do not bring together parents of bullies with parents of targets.
- Increase monitoring of large groups (before and after school, hall passing times, recess, and cafeteria).
- During classes, permit only one student at a time in the restroom; assign a hall monitor to supervise restroom activity and check bathrooms frequently.
- Encourage and expect students and staff to show respect for all students.
- Provide teacher "check-in" support for students who are loners.
- Provide extra monitoring and protection for students who are particularly vulnerable to bullying and harassment because of mental or physical handicapping conditions.

Schoolwide interventions must be carefully planned to target the needs of the school. One suggestion is to elicit feedback from staff and students regarding their concerns. In other words, if bullying is a primary concern among both staff and students, then this behavior would be a primary target for intervention. A behavior checklist at the end of this chapter may be helpful in determining what types of behaviors are problematic and where these behaviors are occurring. Refer to Worksheet 1.1, "Behavior Problems: What, Where, and How Often."

SUGGESTED LEARNING ACTIVITIES
FOR TEACHER AND STAFF TRAINING

- Review Overhead 1.4 at the end of the chapter. Provide teachers with Handout 1.3, "Violence." Discuss strategies to prevent violence at school.
- Review Overhead 1.1 at the end of the chapter to cover main points about bullying. Provide teachers with Handout 1.1, also at the end of the chapter.
- Review Overhead 1.2, "Decrease Bullying by Increasing A.W.A.R.E.N.E.S.S." Using Handout 1.2, cut steps of A.W.A.R.E.N.E.S.S. into nine sections (one for each

letter). Divide teachers and staff into nine groups, giving each group one step. Groups should discuss their step with colleagues for approximately 5 minutes, brainstorming an example of each concept. After 5 minutes one teacher acts as spokesperson for the group, summarizing in 1 minute what they discussed.

- Read the story *Nobody Knew What to Do*. Discuss strategies for decreasing bullying. Share Bibliotherapy Summary 1.1, for the book *Nobody Knew What to Do*, at the end of the chapter.
- Review ideas for classroom activities.
- Model the following lesson plan of a classroom activity; teachers are encouraged to use this activity in their classrooms.

CLASSROOM ACTIVITY: WHO PARTICIPATES IN BULLYING?

Materials needed

Three sheets of large paper labeled "bully," "target," "bystander"
Three markers

Procedure

Discussion: As a class discussion, ask students to define bullying. Introduce the concept of roles involved in bullying interactions: bully, target, and bystander.

Group activity: Divide students into three groups, with each group representing one bullying-related role. In these groups students should brainstorm a list of characteristics they think are common for the role they are assigned. Write characteristics on appropriately labeled large paper. When the groups are finished, review characteristics of each role with the class as a whole.

Group activity: Have the students in each group write a short skit involving each role. Groups then present their skits to the class. After watching the skits, students should identify the roles (i.e., bully, target, or bystander).

Alternate activity: An alternative to having students write skits is to provide prewritten skits for students to role-play. Close by reviewing characteristics and definitions with the class.

Examples of skits
Example 1

BULLY: Student purposely pushes target during lunch and he or she drops his or her tray.

TARGET: Student is pushed by bully and drops lunch tray.

BYSTANDER: Observes the bullying but pretends not to notice.

Example 2: Group of friends are gathered around talking.

BULLY: Did you see what she was wearing today? She looks so stupid!

TARGET: (*Walks up to group just as bully stops talking.*) Hi, guys, how's it going?

BYSTANDERS: (*All act as if they had not heard the rude comments.*)

CLASSROOM ACTIVITY: WHAT IS SEXUAL HARASSMENT?

Objective: Students will learn the definition of sexual harassment and how to respond appropriately.

Caution: Be aware that some students may have been the target and/or perpetrator of sexual harassment. Be honest and direct, but sensitive, when discussing the issues.

Tangled arms game: Refer to Chapter 5, "Teamwork Activities."

Writing activity: Ask students to think about how they felt during the activity. Ask them to write their responses to these questions: "During this activity, how was your personal space affected? Were you comfortable or uncomfortable? Why?"

Pair discussion: After writing their reaction, have students discuss their response with a partner.

Class discussion: Discuss individual responses, calling on volunteers to share their views. Help students recognize that what is comfortable for one person may not be comfortable for another. What is funny to one person may not be funny to someone else, especially if it is hurtful. Explain, "Sometimes others say or do things that make you feel uncomfortable. Name some examples."

Point out that other people might make someone feel uncomfortable by sexually harassing him or her. Ask, "What is sexual harassment?" Show a list containing descriptions of the behaviors that are considered sexual harassment. Refer to Overhead 1.3, "Stop Sexual Harassment." Ask, "If someone hugs you and you don't like it, what could you do?"

Have students brainstorm a list and possibly role play or practice ways to respond to a person who gives "uncomfortable hugs."

Summarize: Underscore the central point for students: If you are being sexually harassed, it is *not* your fault and you *can* get help.

STUDENT RESPONSE TO EMOTIONAL STRESS AND TRAUMA

Individuals vary in the way they respond to stress and trauma. Reactions depend on a number of factors, including age, gender, past history, family support and stability, and the severity of the incident. Another within-child variable often overlooked is that of temperament. Some children are more reactive and excitable by nature, and some are very adaptable; others have difficulty accepting change.

The nature of the trauma also affects the child's or adolescent's response. These factors must be considered:

- Type of trauma
- Amount of time the child was exposed or reexposed to the trauma
- Invasiveness of the trauma to the child's daily life and routine
- Directness or indirectness of exposure to trauma

For instance, if the child saw, heard, and felt the trauma, the effect would likely be much greater than if he or she was indirectly involved, for example, by hearing about the trauma happening to someone else.

Another factor that greatly affects the child's response is the level of control he or she personally had over preventing or escaping trauma. For instance, if the child feels like a passive victim with no power, he or she is much more likely to suffer long-term effects from the trauma. Regaining control is a key issue in helping a child heal. Moving a child from a passive to an active stance empowers him or her. Healing is highly dependent on successfully moving out of the victim role and into a position of personal control.

It is important to understand how individuals respond to trauma and stress. Listed in Table 1.1 are common reactions based on age and developmental maturity.

Assisting younger children who have been exposed to trauma typically includes providing increased support, attention, and nurturing. Keeping a schedule gives the child the security of a routine. Preschool children respond positively to having their physical needs met: provide blankets, food, and drinks. Additionally, children will require extra holding and cuddling from parents and guardians, who may need to make other accommodations for them: Because of sleep problems and nightmares following exposure to trauma, children may want to sleep in close proximity to their parent/guardian; because of heightened fear and anxiety, they may want a light left on in their bedroom.

After a younger child has been traumatized, parents and teachers may find it difficult to deal with his or her behavior problems, which may include angry outbursts, tantrums, screaming, irritability, or aggression toward others. Parents, caretakers, and teachers must be patient. Give the child extra space and time to regain control of his or her behavior. Help the child feel safe by limiting chaotic stimuli and unpredictability. As much as possible, keep things calm and settled in the child's environment.

Elementary school children require many of the same accommodations made for preschool children. However, they are better equipped cognitively to respond to logical rea-

---

TABLE 1.1. Reactions to Stress and Trauma

Note: Look for changes in typical behavior.

All students, regardless of age, may have difficulty with, or changes in, these areas:

- Reverting to immature behaviors
- Complaining of stomachaches and headaches
- Overreacting, jumpy, or easily startled
- Sleeping problems, nightmares, or insomnia
- Change in eating habits
- Angry outbursts of aggressive behavior

Pre-K	Elementary school	Middle and high school
Shivering	Irritable and complaining	Withdrawn and isolated
Crying, irritable, discontent	Excessive fear and anxiety	Excessive fear and anxiety
Sucking thumb	Sadness, crying	Sadness and depression
Wetting, incontinent	Guilt and blaming self	Excessive shame and guilt
Insecure, clinging	Demanding	Careless, risky behaviors
Hyperactive	Attention seeking	Acting out, rebelling
Loud and overreactive	Distractible, daydreamy	Declining grades
	Difficulty concentrating	Change in personality
		Avoidance of feelings
		Self-absorption
		Grotesque humor

soning and to identify and understand their feelings. Although children's explanations for events and situations are commonly based on fantasy and magical thinking, explaining situations in basic terms works well with them by the time they are in elementary school. In addition to emotions of heightened fear, anxiety, and anger, these children are usually dealing with guilt and worry. They need reassurance that they were not the cause of the crisis or trauma. They also need assurance that others are there to support them and that they are not alone.

Adolescents are developing their own identity, and much of that identity is based on what they perceive others are thinking about them. They seek peer approval and support more than younger children. Adolescents are also more aware of their emotions. After experiencing trauma, some may try to avoid emotional pain by participating in high-risk and rebellious behaviors, such as driving dangerously, becoming involved in delinquent activities, taking illicit drugs, drinking alcoholic beverages, shoplifting, or engaging in promiscuous sexual activity. Others turn inward, withdrawing and isolating themselves.

Interventions for adolescents must be based on respect for their need for self-control and independence. Discussing options and answering questions honestly demonstrate respect and assist in building trust. Adolescents respond positively to group support and group activities. Therefore, therapeutic intervention is most effective when the adolescent feels included in a supportive peer group. Reducing isolation is an important step toward emotional healing.

Gender differences in response to trauma become more obvious with age. Boys are less likely than girls to react with crying and hysteria. When dealing with trauma, boys are more likely to make jokes and use irreverent, even grotesque, humor. For instance, in 1993 a fire destroyed the religious compound of Branch Davidian leader David Koresh in Waco, Texas. Approximately 77 men, women, and children died in the fire. The local news carried the story for several weeks. Pictures of the fire and destroyed compound were repeatedly aired on national television. Boys in local schools made jokes about the disaster, such as: "What do the letters W-A-C-O stand for? 'We all cooked ourselves.' " Offended by these insensitive jokes, teachers reprimanded the students. However, teachers and staff need to be patient with adolescents who joke about death and trauma. Although adults may view this behavior as immature, utilizing humor to cope with tragedy is a normal adolescent reaction, particularly for males. This behavior, as well as crying and hysteria, should be viewed as adaptive coping behavior aimed at seeking support and attention during times of stress. Teachers should respond with compassion to this type of humor. An appropriate reaction might include the following statement: "Sometimes we have a difficult time accepting tragedy. We make jokes so we can laugh, because it hurts too much to think about what happened."

All students, no matter what their ages, benefit from a structured and predictable environment. Students look to adults in their lives for stability and security. Daily routines of school are comforting to children and adolescents. Focusing on schoolwork can be a welcome relief from worry and stress. Teachers and other adults in schools must be sensitive to the need for simplicity and predictability. Reduce stress by sticking to routines and making accommodations when necessary.

SUGGESTED READING

American Association of University Women. (2001). *Hostile hallways: Bullying, teasing, and sexual harassment in school.* Washington, DC: Author. (Available from *www.aauw.org*)

Elias, M. J., & Zins, J. E. (Eds.). (2003). *Bullying, peer harassment, and victimization in the schools: The next generation.* New York: Haworth Press.

Garrity, C., Jens, K., Porter, W., Sager, N., & Short-Camilli, C. (2004). *Bully-proofing your elementary school: Teacher's manual and lesson plans* (3rd ed.). Longmont, CO: Sopris West. (Ordering information: Sopris West, ISBN 1-57035-922-9, Product Code: W58683)

Olweus, D. (1993). *Bullying at school: What we know and what we can do.* Malden, MA: Blackwell.

Stein, N., & Sjostrom, L. (1994). *Flirting or hurting? A teachers' guide on student-to-student sexual harassment in schools (grades 6–12).* Washington, DC: National Education Association.

WGBY TV (Producer). (1996). *Flirting or hurting: Sexual harassment in schools* [VHS video]. (Available from GPN, P.O. Box 80669, Lincoln, NE 68501-0669; phone: 800-228-4630, fax: 800-306-2330)

Yoon, J. S., Barton, E., & Taiariol, J. (2004). Relational aggression in middle school: Educational implications of developmental research. *Journal of Early Adolescence, 24,* 303–318.

WEBSITES

www.aauw.org/ef/harass/pdf/completeguide.pdf

Harassment-Free Hallways: How to Stop Sexual Harassment in School: A Guide for Students, Parents, and Schools (2004). You can download this 50-page publication free of charge. The American Association of University Women is a leader in addressing sexual harassment issues.

www.ed.gov/about/offices/list/ocr/checklist.html

This site contains a checklist for addressing harassment in schools. Information and materials are provided by the Office of Civil Rights.

Behavior Problems:
What, Where, and How Often

Source of Feedback: _____ Student, _____ Teacher, _____ Staff

Date: _____

Using the grid below, please describe how frequently these student behaviors occur and where the behaviors are occurring. Use the numbers 1 through 4 to describe the frequency.

1 = not at all this week
2 = once or twice this week
3 = three or four times this week
4 = more than four times this week

	Physical aggression	Verbal aggression	Relational aggression	Conduct problems
Halls				
Classroom				
Cafeteria				
Bathroom				
Recess/Playground				
Before school				
After school				
Walking to school				
Walking home				
Bus				

Types of behavior:

(1) *Physical aggression* includes hitting, kicking, pushing, shoving, pinching, grabbing, scratching, or hurting others.
(2) *Verbal aggression* includes angry yelling, name calling, threatening others, swearing, or using bad words to express anger.
(3) *Relational aggression* includes excluding or leaving someone out on purpose, gossiping to hurt someone's feelings, or telling exaggerated or fabricated stories to hurt someone's reputation. More specifically, students may make statements such as: "I'm not going to be your friend" or "I don't like you."
(4) *Conduct problems* include breaking school rules, ignoring directions from adults, blatantly refusing to follow directions, whining or complaining about school rules, or stealing.

Bullying

Students spend a good portion of their days in school. In order to learn effectively, they need to feel safe and supported. Bullying is a common occurrence in most schools. It is defined as *aggression involving physical, psychological, or sexual harassment that persists over time.* Its negative consequences impact students' ability to learn. Bullying affects the social environment of the school, producing an atmosphere of fear where learning becomes secondary to seeking safety. It is imperative that adults within the school advocate for student safety by being aware of the dynamics of bullying, intervening to stop bullying behaviors, and nurturing individual students.

BULLIES

- Are likely to have been bullied in the past
- Are manipulative, impulsive, and aggressive
- Lack ability to empathize
- Pick on those they believe cannot or will not strike back
- Are often physically stronger than their victims
- Lack constructive problem-solving abilities

WHAT DOES BULLYING LOOK LIKE?

Physical: hitting, pushing, pinching, etc.

Verbal and relational: teasing, ridiculing, vindictive gossip, etc.

BYSTANDERS

Students who reinforce bullying behaviors by watching and doing nothing

TARGETS

- Experience greater depression, anxiety, fear, guilt, shame
- Often feel helpless
- May skip school because they do not feel safe
- May perform worse academically
- Have lower self-esteem
- May run away

TWO TYPES OF VICTIM BEHAVIOR

Passive: lonely, socially rejected, physically weaker, sensitive

Aggressive: hot-tempered, anxious, reactive

WAYS TARGETS COPE

Problem solving: deescalate and resolve problem

Reactive: maintain and intensify problem (more common)

Decreasing Bullying

STAFF TRAINING HANDOUT

Advocate for student safety: Students spend a good portion of their time in school. When students feel safe and supported, they can focus on learning. Bullying is a common occurrence in most schools. Its negative consequences impact students' ability to learn. Bullying affects the social environment of the school, producing an atmosphere of fear where learning becomes secondary to seeking safety. It is imperative that adults within the school advocate for student safety by increasing awareness of bullying behaviors, intervening to stop them, and nurturing individual students.

Watch behavior: School is a social place where students interact with peers. It is essential that school staff pay attention to behavior both in and out of the classroom. Bullies often pick on others when adults are not around. For instance, a girl may bully a smaller boy. He may respond in anger. If the teacher only notices the boy's defensive behavior, he will receive the reprimand. From the teacher's viewpoint, the girl is innocent. Victims are often too scared to say anything. Bullying can be prevented when all adults in the school are on the lookout for inappropriate interactions among students.

Assess seriousness: When a bullying behavior is observed, adults are encouraged to assess how serious the behavior is. Boys often "fight" playfully. Differentiating developmentally appropriate sparring from bullying is essential.

Refer victims and bullies: When a student is bullied, emotional issues are often involved. Both victim and bully may benefit from speaking separately with the mental health professional in the school.

Ensure involvement: In order to bully-proof a school, the entire school community must be involved. From the building administrator to individual students, a united effort to prevent bullying is essential. Parental involvement is also an important aspect of decreasing bullying. As staff, students, and parents work together, bullying can be stopped.

Nurture students: All students need to know that someone cares. Often, those who are hardest to love are the ones who need it most.

Encourage and model appreciation for diversity: Adults can be positive role models in the school. Victims are often socially unaccepted by their peers because of perceived differences. Teachers can model love and acceptance for all students, regardless of their background or personal characteristics. Students must be taught to appreciate diversity and to see diversity as an opportunity to learn rather than a reason to fear.

Share information: Awareness is a major aspect of prevention. As teachers are trained, they can share information with their students in structured lessons. Students can also participate in preparing and teaching classroom skills. As students become aware of bullying and harassment, they are better equipped to recognize and report bullying behaviors. Bullying often occurs outside the range of adult supervision, or in the presence of minimal adult supervision, so increasing supervision adds another dimension to preventing and ending bullying.

Supply social skills training: Many victims and bullies lack appropriate social skills. As social skills are taught in the classroom, teachers can provide opportunities for students to practice the newly learned skills in various contexts, generalizing appropriate behavior across settings. Increased awareness and sensitivity will decrease bullying behaviors.

Violence

The best way to deal with violence is to prevent it from happening. However, when it does occur, there are specific things to remember when dealing with it.

Prevention:

Know the names of students. Greet students each day and get to know them. Talk with them about their interests.

Supervise students. Supervised students have fewer problems with violence. Students should be supervised at all times. Large groups of students with few adults spell trouble. Fights and violence among students occur most frequently in unsupervised or minimally supervised situations.

Be fair and consistent. Follow school rules. Students are more apt to fight when they feel things are not fair or rules are not consistently enforced. School rules provide structure and safety. Know the rules and enforce them. Demonstrate zero tolerance for bullying and teasing.

Listen to students. When you listen, students know you care. When they feel someone is listening and caring, they are less apt to fight.

Be aware. Keep your eyes and ears open. When there are "rumors" of fights, let your supervisor know about your concerns. Let the principal know your worries about students fighting. As much as possible, prevent situations that lead to violence. Know which teachers are trusted by students. Call on these people if you are worried or need help.

Responding to a situation:

If there is a fight, know how to react and what to do.

Do not step in between big students to stop a fight. Although this strategy might work with little kindergarten children, you are likely to get hurt stepping between older, larger students.

Unless properly trained, do not hold/restrain students or try to physically force students apart in a fight.

Eliminate the audience. Direct student onlookers away from the fight; doing so keeps others safe and removes the audience effect.

Be calm. Do not speak loudly. Keep your voice in a normal conversational tone. Remember the "see-saw effect": The louder the student's voice, the softer your voice should be. The faster the student speaks, the slower you should speak.

Call for help immediately. If a student is fighting with, or threatening, another student and there is potential for injury, call the office for help and backup. If you don't have a phone, send a responsible student with a note to the office. Have a "There is trouble—I need assistance" note ready ahead of time. This may be a laminated message you, your supervisor, and principal have prepared ahead of time.

Try to buy some time. Say things such as "I want to hear what you have to say. I am listening. Tell me what the problem is."

Call students by name and let them know that you are there to listen. Encourage the students to step back and talk. Say things such as "I am here to listen. Let's talk this out. I want to hear your side of the story."

Do not threaten students or yell at them.

Don't try to yank, pull, or hold the student. It is almost always best not to touch the student. Stay back and give the student space. Do not get into a power struggle with the student. Do not argue or fight with the student.

BULLYING

Aggression involving physical, psychological, or sexual harassment that persists over time

WHO IS INVOLVED?

- Bullies: Students who seek power and control by physically or verbally attacking those unlikely to strike back

- Targets: Students who are attacked by bullies

- Bystanders: Students who reinforce bullying behaviors by watching and doing nothing

WHAT DOES IT LOOK LIKE?

Physical Aggression—hitting, pushing, pinching, etc.

Relational Aggression—teasing, ridiculing, excluding, mean-spirited gossiping, etc.

WHAT CAN WE DO?

Decrease bullying by increasing A.W.A.R.E.N.E.S.S.

DECREASE BULLYING BY INCREASING
A.W.A.R.E.N.E.S.S.

Advocate for student safety

Watch behavior

Assess seriousness

Refer victims and bullies

Ensure involvement

Nurture students

Encourage appreciation of diversity

Share information

Supply social skills training

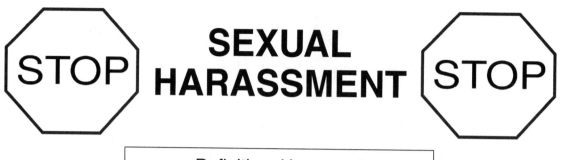

SEXUAL HARASSMENT

Definition: Unwanted
and unwelcome sexual behaviors
considered uncomfortable
and offensive to the target

What it looks like:

- Inappropriate touching
- Groping
- Pinching
- Behavior that is sexually provocative
- Display of pornographic materials

- Sexual comments
- Sexual graffiti
- Sexually oriented jokes
- Sexual gestures
- Sexual bribes

Sexually harassing behavior is **<u>not</u>** a "normal" part of growing up.

VIOLENCE PREVENTION
=
POSITIVE SCHOOL CLIMATE

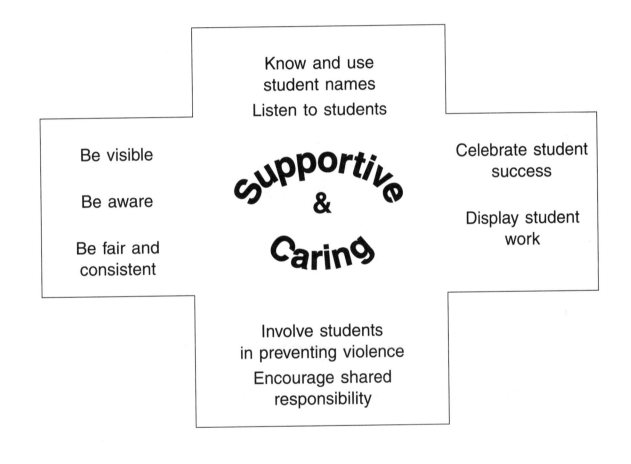

Know and use
student names
Listen to students

Be visible

Be aware

Be fair and
consistent

Supportive
&
Caring

Celebrate student
success

Display student
work

Involve students
in preventing violence
Encourage shared
responsibility

BIBLIOTHERAPY SUMMARY 1.1

Book Title	Nobody Knew What to Do		Excellent	Fair	Poor
Issue Addressed	Bullying	Developmental Level	X		
Author(s)	McCain, Becky Ray	Language and Writing Style	X		
Year of Publication	2001	Quality of Illustrations	X		
Publisher	Albert Whitman & Company	Life Experiences	X		
Address of Publisher	Morton Grove, IL	Portrayal of Problems	X		
ISBN #	0-8075-5711-0	Problem-Solving Process	X		
Price	$14.95	Coping Skills	X		
Age/Grade Level	Ages 4-8	Characterization	X		
# of Pages	21	Dialogue and Communication Skills		X	
Summary of Story: Ray is bullied by classmates. His friend tells the teacher. The teacher and principal step in to make sure the bullying stops. The main message of the book: "Bullying is NEVER OK." (Note: The pictures are excellent.)		Purpose of Emotionally Charged Scenes	X		
		Sensitivity to Human Diversity	X		
		Hope and Support	X		

Suggested Class Activity

After reading the book, role-play the story. Assign students the roles of Ray, good friend, three bystanders, three bullies, teacher, principal, and parent. After the role play, discuss how it makes a person feel when he or she is bullied. On the blackboard, list what to do if students see someone bullying a classmate. Make a poster that says "No Bullying Allowed" to hang on the door of the classroom. Have each person in the class sign the poster to show that he or she will not allow bullying in school.

2

Responding to a Crisis

Melissa Allen Heath, Dawn Sheen, Neil Annandale,
and Bart Lyman

A SCHOOL IN CRISIS

The following story was shared by a school counselor.

"It was a Monday morning in an elementary school. Teachers were coming to work at 7:30, preparing for another week of school, but this week would be different. The principal had died unexpectedly late Sunday evening. Although a few people from the district office had been notified, most teachers entered the school unaware.

"The assistant principal was on the phone making arrangements with the district office crisis team. The school counselor and a few teachers were ushering early arrivals into the teachers' lounge. The talk was direct and quiet. The crisis team would arrive in a few minutes to assist teachers with their classrooms. The teachers and staff, even the stoic custodian, held back tears as they stood in silence. Some were thinking of their students and searching for strategies to explain the death of Ms. Hutchings. Others were numb, thinking random thoughts and finding it difficult to concentrate. It was going to be a long and intense day.

"The school's roster listed 646 students. School started at 8:00. Students on the early bus would arrive in just a few minutes. Who would be in charge? Ms. Hutchings always greeted everyone on the intercom. She was always there. Every morning for the past 8 years she greeted students as they entered the building. To the students, she

Neil Annandale, MA, Graduate Student in Counseling Psychology, Brigham Young University, Provo, Utah.

23

was as much a part of the building as the flagpole or drinking fountain. Now she was gone.

"Although the school was prepared for a fire drill—everyone could file out of the building in 3 minutes and 22 seconds—the school had never prepared for the sudden death of their principal. This elementary school was not prepared to deal with such a shock. Everything was in slow motion. Nothing felt real. Everything was out of sync; the familiarity of daily routine had been pulled out from under us. Our school was not the same.

"As promised, the district crisis team arrived at 8:00. They brought handouts on grief and death for teachers to use in their classrooms. Handouts were helpful. It comforted teachers to have a piece of paper with information. They appreciated knowing what was expected of them, what to say, and what to do.

"Even today, 7 years since that dreadful Monday morning, teachers and staff still remember the overwhelming feeling of responsibility. The district crisis team could not get to all the students and adults who needed help. At the end of the day, everyone was emotionally exhausted. There was a feeling of emptiness as the last student left the building."

WHAT IS A SCHOOL CRISIS PLAN?

Chaos created by a school crisis, if unchecked, undermines school safety, security, and stability. To counter chaos and instability, a crisis plan provides an emergency protocol to structure and organize staff responsibilities and available resources. The purpose of the plan is to provide order and stability by pulling the school community together.

An effective crisis plan relies on all members of the team and all parts of the plan working together effectively. A well-defined crisis plan requires two basic components: preparation and follow-through. Preparation is based on predetermining effective steps and strategies to take following an "incident." Preparation also includes adequately training staff to follow these steps in the event of a crisis. Follow-through hinges on trained staff actually putting their training into practice and following the crisis plan's prescribed steps.

All schools are required to have a fire-escape plan. Additionally, most crisis plans include protocol for the following incidents: suicide, death, grief and loss, violence and aggression, weapon on campus, threat of violence, school shooting, gang activity, natural disaster, bomb scare, illicit drug use, abuse (sexual and physical), community or national disaster, medical emergency, campus intruder, and so on.

Getting down to basic information, a crisis plan anticipates "What if . . . ? Then this." It organizes people and resources, defines duties and lines of authority, and reduces panic and chaos. With proper training of staff, a good plan instills confidence with its three-phase timeline of crisis intervention: prevention, immediate intervention during the crisis, and postvention services for those needing support after the initial crisis.

Ideally, crisis plans should be user-friendly, accessible and familiar to all, realistic, and tailored to individual school settings. Tailoring crisis plans includes considering potential language and communication barriers, accounting for diverse needs of students and community, and effectively utilizing varied resources and strengths of school personnel. Crisis plans should be flexible and adaptable to the changing needs of students, schools, and communities.

COMMON PROBLEMS WITH CRISIS PLANS

Problems arise when crisis plans are not an integral part of the school's daily operations. Even though well intentioned, those formulating plans at the district level do not know specific details about each school in the district. Some of these details include the physical layout of buildings, entrance and exit routes to schools, skills of staff members, characteristics and diversity of school communities, communication needs, accessibility to community services, and strengths and weaknesses in school leadership.

Teachers and staff may have a false sense of security with nothing more than a district crisis plan in place. Although aware of the district crisis plan, they have no idea where they fit into it or what would actually happen in the event of a schoolwide crisis. Unfortunately, if adults in the school are not invested in the plan and are not trained appropriately, the plan's effectiveness is greatly reduced. When a schoolwide crisis occurs, teachers and staff who do not know what to do inadvertently increase the chaos and panic. Students sense leaders' confusion and insecurity. There is no anchor of stability and support. This vacuum places students and the entire school in a very vulnerable position.

Schools must become proactive in their efforts to create a crisis plan that fits their needs. Even when a district plan is in place, the individual school must tailor and adapt that plan. Additionally, the school must make a backup plan in the event that the district crisis team is not immediately available. This does not mean that schools must start from scratch to develop a totally new plan. On the contrary, it is recommended that schools review district plans and only make necessary accommodations or adaptations.

In developing, modifying, and updating a school crisis plan, several individuals representing all levels of personnel within the school must be included. From top leadership to supportive services, everyone must take an active part in discussing the needs of the school. Each person has a different perspective, depending on his or her level of training, responsibility, and experience.

Plans must be in a format that is easily accessed and understood. All teachers and staff members must have a crisis plan made available to them. Additionally all adults must receive basic training concerning their duties. Ongoing discussion throughout the school year keeps the crisis plan in a "ready" position and heightens awareness of being prepared.

One problem that requires ongoing attention is keeping crisis plans updated. If there is no grass-roots effort within the school to keep plans current, problems arise when outdated information compromises crisis intervention. Phone trees, in particular, are useless if not continually updated. However, this problem is easily remedied if a secretary is assigned responsibility to keep the phone tree updated.

WHAT IS A CRISIS TEAM?

A crisis team consists of individuals organized to work together as a unit and carry out designated duties listed in the crisis plan. The core team typically consists of school mental health professionals supported by community professionals, teachers, and school staff. Two levels of crisis teams may operate within the school: a district-level team and a school-based team. Crisis teams consider two basic student needs: physical and emotional well-being.

Specific duties listed in crisis plans should be assigned to specific individuals based on their abilities and skills in relation to crisis intervention. Meeting the needs of students and families during a crisis requires a variety of abilities. Are teachers, staff, and administrators trained in emergency medical procedures, such as CPR and first aid? Who speaks languages represented in the community? Who has strong communication skills and conflict resolution skills to assist in deescalating volatile situations? Who remains calm in the midst of chaos?

When assigning duties to individuals, it is important to consider not only their abilities and professional training in regard to crisis intervention but also their level of responsibility, availability, and familiarity with students and the school. Crisis intervention duties require varying levels of responsibility and accountability. Control is a key issue during a crisis. Who is in control of students? To whom do the students look for direction? Typically, in a school setting the principal is the key figure holding the highest position of power. Teachers hold power under the principal's lead. Crisis plans that utilize the existing hierarchy of power within schools are more likely to be effective and efficient during critical incidents.

In addition to responsibility and accountability, availability must also be considered when organizing crisis teams and assigning duties. Who is most likely to be with students when a crisis occurs? Who can get to the site quickly? Availability is a primary reason for involving teachers and school staff in all aspects of crisis plans. Teachers are with students. Realistically speaking, teachers and staff will most likely be the ones handling problems and crises as they arise.

Another important factor to consider in organizing crisis teams and setting plans in place is selecting individuals familiar with students and the school. Who is a familiar and trusted face? Who knows how to function in a school setting? Who knows the layout of the school? Who is familiar with school policy and power structure?

More specifically, the unique needs of school and community must be considered when organizing district-level crisis teams. Such teams should represent the cultures and languages of families they serve. Individuals with language skills who are able and willing should be invited to serve as interpreters on the crisis team. With adequate preparation and supervision, all school staff members, including paraeducators, are potential candidates.

Possible barriers to providing services during a crisis must be considered. Examples of barriers may include a limited number of trained professionals, particularly those who have formed ties with minority groups; limited financial resources; lack of interpreters to communicate with non-English-speaking populations; difficulties in quickly contacting parents due to the transient nature of some families; inconsistent or nonexistent phone services in homes; and limited access to transportation.

CONTROL AND ORGANIZATION DURING A SCHOOL CRISIS

Organizing people and resources is the most important function of a crisis plan. In particular, large-scale incidents require an organized hierarchy of command. The Incident Command System (ICS) identifies five major areas of organization: management, planning/ intelligence, operations, logistics, and finance administration (Johnson, 2000). In the school system, principals typically head management and are seen as the top person in the chain of command. Also involved in management are campus security officers and media spokespersons.

Teachers and staff are typically involved with planning/intelligence and operations. These functions include gathering information regarding critical incidents or emergency situations, documenting and sharing information with the principal or campus security officer, and assisting with emergency response. Teachers and staff assist with on-the-spot student needs, medical emergencies, and evacuating students or assisting with lockdown procedures.

The custodian or support staff (secretaries, cafeteria workers, and office aides) may assist the principal or administrator with the logistics function of ICS by helping to organize materials and supplies and providing other crisis workers with the supplies/resources they need to perform their duties. They lock or unlock doors, provide students and crisis team members with food and drinks, and assist in setting up group counseling or debriefing rooms. Other duties may include running errands for supplies, assisting with cleanup, gathering and collecting emergency materials, and so on.

CLASSROOM EMERGENCY KITS

Teachers can also assist by preparing an emergency box and backpack for their classroom. Each teacher should thoughtfully prepare for the specific needs of his or her class. A box might contain a first-aid kit, several blankets/sheets, and emergency food and water. Each teacher should also prepare an emergency backpack to use in case of evacuation. The backpack might be stocked with a flashlight, basic first-aid kit, class roll with updated phone numbers and contact information (in a protective plastic sheet), granola bars, several bottles of water, favorite children's book (for younger children), whistle, tablet, pencil, pen, and a walkie-talkie or cell phone. Another suggestion is to include two laminated sheets of colored paper: a green piece of paper to signal the principal from a distance that all their students are accounted for, and a red piece of paper to indicate a missing student or a need for assistance.

ROLES AND RESPONSIBILITIES OF EACH ADULT

When teachers and staff think of their role in a crisis, they think of fire drills. Basically everyone knows how to exit the building in case of a fire. Unfortunately, other than exiting the building, most teachers and staff are unaware of their school's crisis plan. Although most plans depend heavily on district crisis teams in the event of a major catastrophe, all teachers and staff should familiarize themselves with the crisis plan specific to their school.

However, even when crisis plans are made available to teachers and staff, training is not typically provided to teach and inform them of their duties, as well as how to perform those duties. Crisis plans are frequently viewed as someone else's responsibility. Untrained and uninformed, teachers and staff do not feel confident in assisting. When a crisis does occur, they look to others for help and direction. They have no idea how they could assist in a crisis. They think crisis plans are for crisis teams. This perception must change. Each adult in the school must participate in crisis prevention and intervention.

Ideally, all school employees and volunteers should be prepared to assist with crisis intervention. With appropriate training, each adult in the school can provide emotional support to students, preventing or lessening the effects of crisis. At every level of crisis intervention, more effort must be invested in preparing individuals within schools, particularly staff who work directly with students.

On a day-to-day basis teachers and support staff are on the front lines dealing with students' emotional needs. Teachers and staff must know what to say and what to do in order to provide immediate and appropriate emotional support. When offering assistance to students in crisis, there are basic instructions (refer to Overhead 2.1, "Crisis Response Skills: Lend a Helping Hand," at the end of this chapter). On the palm is the first and foremost duty to foster during a crisis: *Stay calm.* Staying calm helps an individual to think clearly and talk softly and slowly. Students depend on adults as their anchor of security and stability.

Adults must also reassure, listen, observe, report, and control.

- *Reassure*: "I'm here for you, I care. We are in this together."
- *Listen*: Listen more than talk.
- *Observe*: Observe behaviors; gather and document information.
- *Report*: For serious matters (extreme behaviors, safety issues, abuse, and suicidal comments), report concerns to supervisors/professionals.
- *Control*: Stay in control, do not panic, know your role and take responsibility for it.

Each teacher and staff member must know where he or she fits into the chain of command. Review the crisis plan and determine which duties apply to you. Clarify these duties with your supervisor or administrator. Typically staff and teachers are involved in four major areas of responsibility:

- *Escaping to safety.* Exiting the building (e.g., fire drill).
- *Staying in the building.* Seeking shelter in the building (lockdown).

- *Keeping students safe and calm*. Assisting with immediate needs, reducing chaos, keeping order.
- *Communicating*. Providing information about students' needs to supervisors and administrators, listening for directions from principal and professionals, and communicating with students and parents.

Role plays are helpful in practicing desired skills to prepare staff and teachers to assist with crisis intervention. A suggested outline for teaching crisis skills by using role play follows:

1. Present basic information.
2. Model behavior by live demonstration or a video clip.
3. Set up a scenario.
4. Role-play and practice skills.
5. Share constructive feedback.
6. Process information and discuss.
7. Summarize main points, check for understanding.

A CRISIS PLAN IN ACTION

The following story, shared by a teacher, illustrates one school's crisis plan in action.

"It was a cold November day. Third hour had just begun as students took out pencil and paper to take a pop quiz. Suddenly, they were saved by the bell. An unexpected fire alarm was sounded. It wasn't a scheduled drill, and I wondered if I should ignore it or act. Relying on previous trainings, I expertly instructed students to go outside and line up in our preassigned location. One student grabbed our white emergency bucket with the bright pink paper flag proclaiming our room number. As we entered the hall, we fought to find a place among the mass of students being herded toward the doors.

"Cool air hit our faces as we stepped outside. Bright pink paper flags lined up next to each other in numerical order, with the students belonging to each room standing behind them. Although I would like to say that each student was perfectly behaved, standing docilely in line, this was not the case. Curious, social eighth graders tried to leave their classes to find friends, who had no more knowledge than they did about the situation. Teachers struggled to keep control of the chaos and confusion.

"Each teacher opened his or her bucket and pulled out what they hoped was a current class list. Students were accounted for, and a student runner took the message to Command Center (marked by a bright pink flag with 'Command Center' printed in big, bold letters).

"As a teacher, it is important to remain calm in crisis situations. Students clustered around me, asking if I knew what was going on. Other students came to the circle, proclaiming that their best friend's second cousin's parent's favorite pet's owner had told them there really was a fire that had burned down the other side of the school. Smoke billowed in the air, seemingly confirming the rumors. I did my best to dispel the rumor by reassuring students that we would be informed of the facts when this information became available.

"In the meantime, students began jumping up and down in an effort to stay warm as the cool autumn air penetrated their clothing. Thinking quickly, I began to shout out commands in French. My students were soon engaged in running, jumping, turning, pointing, and singing (much to their peers' enjoyment and their own embarrassment). One thing missing from my white emergency bucket was something entertaining to keep students occupied. They were soon bored of responding to my commands, so I assigned a student to be in charge of a stirring game of 'Pierre Dit,' French for 'Simon Says.'

"While occupied with the game, I noticed several of my students were shivering, clothed in summer shorts and T-shirts. They looked nearly frozen. Luckily, as we were exiting the classroom, I had grabbed a stray sweatshirt and blanket stacked next to my desk. Several students borrowed these from me and huddled together.

"Looking around, I saw my department head standing a few feet away, talking to another teacher in the department. As she finished, she came to me and informed me that a classroom on the other side of the school had caught fire, but it was under control. We were just waiting for the fire marshal to come and let us know what would happen next. She instructed me to keep students as busy as possible until we knew if we would be sending them home or not.

"I interrupted the game of 'Pierre Dit' to share the latest news with my students. Excitement rippled through the class upon hearing that they might get to go home early. Nearly an hour had passed since the initial sounding of the fire alarm. Students were bored and beginning to get hungry as lunch hour approached. I gave students an assignment to write five sentences in French about what they were feeling. Sharing pencils and paper from the emergency bucket, each student quickly completed the assignment, anticipating some type of reward. Luckily, my white bucket contained enough small candies to reward each student.

"Students got colder and hungrier as time passed. Teachers were given frequent updates on the situation as members of the crisis team, armed with walkie-talkies, circulated among us. With each update, students became more excited as it was beginning to look like they would be going home early. Finally, we were instructed to move our students around the Command Center, where the vice-principal was standing on his white bucket and holding a megaphone. He outlined the situation for students, dispelling any rumors they might have heard. Only one classroom had sustained serious damage, but smoke had gotten into the heating ducts of the school, and the fire marshal had declared it unsafe for anyone to be in the building. Cheers erupted as he announced they would be going home for the day.

"Once students were quiet again, he outlined what was expected of them. Classes would be dismissed one by one to go into the school quickly and obtain necessary items from the classroom (e.g., house keys). Students were expected to take a specific route through the building; they were told not to go into any other part of the school.

Buses would line up in front of the school. Teachers were responsible for accounting for each student, making sure each student either boarded a bus or had a way home. Parents were being notified on all major radio stations in the area to meet their students on the opposite end of the school from where the buses were loading. (There was a department store with a large parking lot where parents could park while waiting.) Secretaries were notifying parents by utilizing the phone tree.

"As students were dismissed, we walked quickly to the classroom and through the school to the buses. One of my students looked at me and said, 'My parents are out of town, and I'm staying with my grandparents. They only live a block away. Can I walk there?' I looked at him and said, 'You're only wearing shorts and a T-shirt! You'll freeze to death!' He returned my gaze and rolling his eyes said, 'I just stood outside for 2 hours. I think I'll be fine.' What could I say? He was right. I made a permission note, listing who he was and where he was going, and sent him on his way. Students boarded the buses or found their parents and safely went home.

"As I reentered the school, a crisis team member was standing by the door. The fire marshal wasn't clear about how long the school would be unsafe. Phone trees would be utilized the following morning to let us know if we could come to school. We would be debriefed later at an emergency faculty meeting. Teachers were exhausted and grateful for a half day off. That night, I opened the newspaper to find the school on the front page. The journalist described the scene in detail, including the pink shirt and khaki pants the principal was wearing.

"The next school day, as the principal talked to the students about what had happened, he made sure to let everyone know that his shirt was salmon-colored and the pants weren't khaki, they were expensive suit pants. The publicity surrounding the principal's pink shirt made for great jokes at future faculty meetings.

"Several months later, our principal had a birthday. Four days before his birthday, the vice-principal announced to students that he wanted to let the principal know how much we cared. They were asked to honor their principal by wearing pink on his birthday. The day arrived and the halls were a great sea of pink. Students were united in celebrating his birth. The day of the fire was long, and repairing the school was costly, but the unity gained through the experience was priceless."

EFFECTIVE CRISIS INTERVENTION FOR STUDENTS FROM DIVERSE BACKGROUNDS

Meeting the unique needs of students in crisis requires sensitivity and skill when planning and adapting services. Sensitivity to individual characteristics, strengths, and needs is based on an understanding of human diversity and cultural and societal influences. This understanding directly influences our perception of how a crisis affects an individual or group, how we identify problems, and how we intervene with students and families in crisis. The following incident demonstrates the significant challenges in providing crisis intervention to culturally diverse students.

The Stockton Schoolyard Shootings

On January 17, 1989, the Stockton, California, schoolyard shootings brought international attention to the devastation and chaos created by a school tragedy, including the lack of culturally sensitive services available to a diverse community (Armstrong, 1991). During morning recess, a man carrying a semiautomatic AK-47 rifle randomly shot at groups of children on the playground, killing five students. A teacher and 29 students were also wounded in the attack. The incident occurred at Cleveland Elementary School, a campus serving approximately 970 students, of whom almost 70% were of Southeast Asian descent. The majority of students' parents were non-English-speaking.

Armstrong, the school psychologist assigned to Cleveland Elementary, described the confusion of frightened parents rushing onto the school grounds trying desperately to locate their children. Because of the language barrier, communicating with parents was difficult. The panic escalated as parents realized police and emergency medical crews were transporting unidentified children to the hospital. For several hours, parents were uncertain if their children were safe, missing, injured, or dead. For mental health professionals in the school and the community, this tragic incident created the overwhelming challenge of providing emergency mental health services to an ethnically, culturally, and linguistically diverse school and community.

James and Gilliland state that "although crisis intervention is never easy, cultural insensitivity may make it even more difficult" (2001, p. 26). Moreover, Romualdi and Sandoval (1995) assert that "communities most in need of services often include a high concentration of ethnically and culturally diverse students and families. Service provision, as a result, must be culturally appropriate and reflect growing population trends" (p. 309).

CURRENT SCHOOL DEMOGRAPHICS

Ethnic Diversity

The changing demographics in North American schools highlight the increasing need for cultural sensitivity in providing appropriate emotional first aid for students. The National Center for Educational Statistics (NCES, 2002) reported that during the 2000–2001 school year, approximately 40% of the 47 million children and youth enrolled in public education in the United States comprised students of color: 17% African American, 16% Hispanic, 4% Asian/Pacific Islander, and 1% Native American/Alaska Native. Students of color outnumber European American students in six states (California, Hawaii, Louisiana, Mississippi, New Mexico, and Texas), and many urban areas such as Washington, DC, currently report that minority students outnumber European American students (NCES, 2002).

In sharp contrast to student diversity, a large majority of teachers (84%) are European American. Only 9.9% of teachers are African American and 5.4% are Hispanic (U.S. Census Bureau, 2002). A national shortage of minority teachers is particularly evident in special education, which employs 9.7% African American, and only 2.4% Hispanic teachers (U.S. Census Bureau). Even more striking than the ethnic mismatch between student and teacher populations is the fact that almost 95% of school psychologists are European

American (Curtis, Grier, Abshier, Sutton, & Hunley, 2002; Curtis, Hunley, Walker, & Baker, 1999).

Linguistic Diversity

Further compounding the complexity of meeting students' diverse needs is the fact that almost 9 million school-age children—17% of all U.S. students—speak a language other than English in the home (U.S. Census Bureau, 2001). California and Texas have a particularly high proportion of linguistic diversity. For example, based on the 2000–2001 language census, one-fourth of California's 6.1 million students speak a language other than English in the home.

During the 2000–2001 school year across the nation, only one-third of the needed "English learning" teacher positions as filled with appropriately trained and certified specialists (National Center for Educational Statistics, 2002). The National Association of School Psychologists (NASP) report that, similar to the shortage of teachers with expertise in language skills, only 10% of the association's members are fluent in a language other than English (Curtis et al., 1999).

Providing services to students who speak a language other than English is further complicated by the ever-increasing number of languages spoken. In Chicago, students in public schools represent approximately 200 languages (Bracken & McCallum, 1998; Pasko, 1994). Examples of other urban school districts with over 50 languages represented in the student body include Palm Beach, Florida; Tempe, Arizona; Plano, Texas; Des Plaines, Illinois; and Knoxville, Tennessee (Bracken & McCallum).

MATCHING SERVICES TO MULTICULTURAL NEEDS

Cultural sensitivity must be applied to all areas of service provision, including crisis intervention. In providing services to children and families in crisis, cultural sensitivity and awareness of diverse needs are particularly important. Recognizing and tailoring crisis intervention to fit the needs of diverse student populations will positively impact the quality of services provided in schools and communities.

In order to provide effective and sensitive emotional first aid to students of diverse backgrounds, mental health providers, teachers, staff, and administrators must take responsibility for increasing their personal awareness and understanding of student diversity issues and concerns. Those responsible for school crisis plans must consider and incorporate their community's diverse characteristics and needs during the formulation stage.

Understanding the unique needs of students requires a basic knowledge of how children and adolescents function in relation to their peers, school, family, community, and world. Sue and Sue (2003) use a diagram of three concentric circles to describe a tripartite framework for understanding the development of personal identity. The innermost circle represents the individual level, comprised of those characteristics unique to the person, such as his or her genetic makeup and specific life experiences. The next level, the group level, includes the similarities among people who share the "social, cultural, and political distinctions made in our society" (p. 13). The final, universal, level is composed of the commonalities that exist among all human beings.

The group level of personal identity is of particular importance in understanding the implications of cultural diversity. Sue and Sue (2003, p. 7) explain that, through socialization, participation in cultural groups can "exert a powerful influence over us and influence our worldviews," shaping the way that situations and events are perceived and interpreted. In the National Strategy for Suicide Prevention, culture is defined as "the integrated pattern of human behavior that includes thoughts, communication, actions, customs, beliefs, values, and institutions of a racial, ethnic, faith, or social group" (U.S. Department of Health and Human Services, 2001, p. 197).

In addition to understanding the definition of cultural diversity, becoming knowledgeable about changing demographics in U.S. schools and, more importantly, in individual schools and communities heightens cultural awareness in planning and providing effective crisis intervention. Acquiring this knowledge can be accomplished by annually reviewing the NCES (*nces.ed.gov/*), which provides accurate up-to-date information on the breakdown of ethnic and language diversity nationally and by state. Information is also readily available from local school districts, which can provide a quick overview of local diversity, on both a district and individual school level. Schools typically provide the public with school district statistics, including percentages of "free and subsidized school lunches" and language and ethnic breakdowns.

PLANNING AND CONDUCTING A MULTICULTURAL NEEDS ASSESSMENT

A second step involved in tailoring crisis intervention to culturally diverse populations is to conduct a needs assessment of the school and community. Responding to specific populations in a personalized manner requires knowing their needs and their resources. A needs assessment may include, but is not limited to, the following questions:

What languages are spoken in the school and in students' homes?
What cultures are represented in the school district?
How do people from these cultures cope with crisis?
What are their natural coping skills?
What resources currently exist and which organizations can be called upon and utilized during a crisis?

An additional but often overlooked variable to consider is the diversity of spiritual and religious beliefs. Belief systems hold important implications for how families perceive a crisis, how they choose to deal with it, and most importantly, how they seek and accept assistance from mental health professionals. Commenting on the importance of understanding belief systems and the spiritual needs of those in crisis, Pedersen (2003) reported on the devastation caused by the earthquakes that hit Taiwan during the 1999–2000 year and survivors' attitudes toward crisis counselors. Though crisis mental health services were available, there was not a demand for counseling intervention. In fact, Pedersen stated that victims were "not interested in counseling" and, in fact, saw "talk therapy" as "making the problem worse" (p. 397). Rather than seeking or accepting professional counseling services, survivors were in need of Buddhist priests to conduct ceremonies resolving spiritual issues surrounding the death of family members. Suffice it to say that, in advance of a crisis, alternatives to traditional mental health services must be considered, explored, and accessed.

Mental health providers can suggest changes in the organizational structure for providing intervention once they recognize the specific differences in how individuals from diverse backgrounds perceive and deal with crisis. Understanding the uniqueness of cultural backgrounds and tailoring interventions to compliment natural support systems of family, friends, and community will create better services and healthier, more productive, outcomes.

STAFF TRAINING ACTIVITY: SENSITIVITY TO STUDENT DIVERSITY

Staff members can discuss the information from Handout 2.1, "Diversity in Our Schools" (at the end of the chapter), and compare their school's statistics with the national statistics on student diversity. The goal is to equip all staff members with the ability to answer these questions:

- "What is the ethnic breakdown of students in our school district?"
- "How many languages are spoken in our school district?"
- "What are the religious beliefs represented in our school district? How could our school involve ministers and clergy to assist with crisis intervention?"
- "In case of emergency, how would our school contact parents who do not have telephones?"
- "In regard to crisis intervention, how can our school make accommodations for students from diverse backgrounds? Identify some unique needs of students and families in our school and community."

STAFF TRAINING ACTIVITY: REVIEWING YOUR SCHOOL'S CRISIS PLAN

Purpose: To familiarize staff members with their school's crisis plan.

Suggestion: Invite a member of the district crisis team or someone who is responsible for the school crisis plan to assist with this staff activity.

Materials for each person

Pencil and paper
Handout 2.2, "Questions about Your School Crisis Plan" (at the end of the chapter)
School crisis plan

If possible, provide all participants with a copy of the crisis plan. If this is not possible, provide each group (below) with a copy of the crisis plan.

Instructions

- Break into groups of five.
- Provide each group with pencils, paper, school crisis plan, and Handout 2.2.
- Read these directions aloud: "Answer the questions on the sheet identified as 'Questions about Your School Crisis Plan' [Handout 2.2]. Each question is worth 1 point. Double the points if you know the answer to a question without referring to your school crisis plan. The group earning the most points wins the game. You have 15 minutes to complete this activity."
- Determine which group has earned the most points and announce the winner. Discuss the correct answers.
- Summarize: "It is important to have a basic understanding of your school crisis plan. Know your responsibilities and how your role fits into the crisis plan."

Assignment: "Highlight information in the crisis plan that applies to you."

STAFF TRAINING ACTIVITY: ROLE-PLAYING CRISIS SCENARIOS

Purpose: To provide opportunities for problem solving. Role plays help staff members think through their individual responsibilities and what they would do in case of student emergencies. This activity also familiarizes staff with the school's crisis plan.

Materials for each person

Pencil and paper
Handout 2.3, "Role-Playing Crisis Scenarios" (at the end of the chapter)
School crisis plan

If possible, provide all participants with a copy of the crisis plan. If this is not possible, provide each group (below) with a copy of the crisis plan.

Instructions

- Break into groups of five (role-playing in smaller groups is more comfortable for participants).
- Provide each group with pencils, paper, school crisis plan, and copies of Handout 2.3.
- Read these directions aloud: "Read the role-play scenario. Although you are provided with some information, the information is limited. Assign parts and role-play for 2 minutes. It does not have to be perfect. After the role play, discuss the choices

that were made. Identify three things that went well, and identify one thing that was particularly difficult in the role play. What makes a situation like this tough to handle?"

- Review the questions listed at the end of each role play.

Following the role plays, summarize: "It is important to have a basic understanding of your school crisis plan. Know your responsibilities and how they fit into the crisis plan."

Assignment: "Review your school's crisis plan. List your responsibilities in helping with the following situations: school lockdown, helping a student who is upset and crying, responding to a student's suicidal comments, and reporting abuse."

The following information will assist the instructor with the discussions following each role play.

Note: During crisis situations you typically do not have the luxury of time. The role plays in this exercise are designed to give you an opportunity to "think on your feet," problem solve, and experience the immediacy and intensity of feelings associated with crisis situations.

Role Play 1: You are the secretary for an elementary school. You are talking with a student (Tami) who was recently in an automobile accident (3 weeks ago). Although Tami suffered only minor injuries, the father and younger sister were seriously injured and died soon after the accident. The student is in the office crying. Role-play how you would respond to this situation. Consider the following questions:

- *What information is missing from this scenario that would influence your response?* The student's age is an important factor to consider. Other factors affecting your response as a helper include how well you know the student and situational factors such as what triggered her crying. It is also important to consider the time of day. If this is at the end of the day, you should also think about getting the student ready to go home safely. If the incident occurred at the beginning of the day, you would consider helping the student return to class.

- *How busy/noisy is the office area?* You may be very busy answering the phone and helping other students and teachers. As the secretary, you must understand that it is OK to ask the counselor or other available adult to assist. A student who is upset and crying may feel overwhelmed by the lack of privacy and embarrassed by others asking them "What's wrong?" On the other hand, the student may enjoy extra attention in the busy office area.

- *What strategies could you use to calm this student?* Listening to Tami is important. Let her know that she is not alone, that you are there for her. Use the basic listening skills discussed in Chapter 4.

- *If Tami settles down, stops crying, and goes back to class, would you still need to tell anyone about her visit to the office?* It is important to keep the teacher and counselor updated on Tami's needs.

- *What would you do if Tami did not calm down and stop crying?* It is not your responsibility to solve Tami's problem. You can assist by listening and showing support for her, but for more serious problems, your responsibility is to refer her—or any student in a similar situation—to the counselor.

• *Would you refer this student to the school's mental health professional (counselor, social worker, or school psychologist)?* Refer Tami if the crying is intense or if she needs additional assistance beyond what you can offer. Always keep the counselor and teacher updated on your observations of students who are at risk for emotional difficulties.

Role Play 2: You are a teacher at the middle school. It is 3:00 (right after the junior high bell rings to release students). Three friends of a 14-year-old girl come into your class-room and tell you that they are concerned about Jessica because she told them that she "did not think life was worth living any more." They say Jessica has progressively become more withdrawn and sad over the last month. As a teacher, what would you do? Consider the following questions:

• *What advice should you, as the teacher, give to Jessica's friends?* It is important for friends to be supportive of each other, but for something this serious, adults need to help. The friends should be commended for expressing their concerns to an adult. Tell the students that you will talk with the counselor and call Jessica's parent/guardian. Let them know how lucky Jessica is to have such great friends. Also let them know that when some-one is as depressed as Jessica, he or she may need more help than friends can give. It is important that you check back with Jessica's friends during the week. Ask the counselor to meet with the friends and provide support for them, if needed.

• *Does the school crisis plan tell teachers what to do when a student makes suicidal statements?* Read the school crisis plan to determine what is appropriate to do in this type of situation. If the plan does not include this important information, talk with the school's mental health professional and clarify what teachers and staff should do when a student talks about suicide.

• *Do you have a positive relationship with Jessica and her parent/guardian? Are parent/guardian emergency phone numbers available in the office?* When teachers and parents have a good relationship, it is much easier to call parents when problems arise. Teachers can be supportive in encouraging parents to seek professional help for students. Parents must always be notified when there are concerns about a student's safety.

• *Can you contact the school's mental health professional and express concerns?* Mental health professionals in the school provide support during difficult situations such as this. When teachers hear or learn of students making suicidal comments, they must always express their concerns to the counselor. If the counselor is not in the building, teachers should report their concerns to the principal. Suicidal comments require immediate atten-tion. Suicidal comments should NEVER be discounted.

• *What should you do if the student has already left the school?* You should check to see if the mental health professional is still in the building. This is a serious problem requiring immediate attention. If the counselor or school psychologist is not in the build-ing, you should follow directions given in your school's crisis plan. There may be an emer-gency number listed in the crisis plan. (Emergency numbers are also listed in the phone book.) As soon as possible, inform the parent/guardian about the student's comments.

SUGGESTED READING

Athey, J., & Moody-Williams, J. (2003). *Developing cultural competence in disaster mental health programs: Guiding principles and recommendations*. Rockville, MD: U.S. Department of Health and Human Services.

Brock, S. E., Sandoval, J., & Lewis, S. (2001). *Preparing for crisis in the schools: A manual for building school crisis response teams* (2nd ed.). New York: Wiley.

Canter, A. S., & Carroll, S. A. (Eds.). (1999). *Crisis prevention and response: A collection of NASP resources*. Bethesda, MD: National Association of School Psychologists.

Johnson, K. (2000). *School crisis management: A hands-on guide to training crisis response teams* (2nd ed.). Alameda, CA: Hunter House.

Pitcher, G. D., & Poland, S. (1992). *Crisis intervention in the schools*. New York: Guilford Press.

Poland, S., Pitcher, G., & Lazarus, P. J. (1999). Best practices in crisis intervention. In A. S. Canter & S. A. Carroll (Eds.), *Crisis prevention and response: A collection of NASP resources* (pp. 69–86). Bethesda, MD: National Association of School Psychologists.

WEBSITE

nces.ed.gov/

National Center for Education Statistics (NCES).

Diversity in Our Schools

Ethnic Diversity of Students:

40% of U.S. students are students of color.

- 17% African American
- 16% Hispanic
- 4% Asian/Pacific Islander
- 1% Native American/Alaska Native

Students of color outnumber European American students in six states: California, Hawaii, Louisiana, Mississippi, New Mexico, and Texas.

Ethnic Diversity of Teachers:

- 84% European American
- 9.9% African American
- 5.4% Hispanic

Ethnic Diversity of Teachers in Special Education:

- 87% European American
- 9.7% African American
- 2.4% Hispanic

Ethnic Diversity of School Mental Health Providers:

- 95% of school psychologists are European American
- 10% speak another language

Linguistic Diversity of Students:

Students speaking a language other than English in the home:
- 17% of U.S. students
- 25% of California's students

Number of Languages in Schools:

- 200 in Chicago schools
- 50+ languages in Palm Beach, Florida; Tempe, Arizona; Plano, Texas; Des Plaines, Illinois; and Knoxville, Tennessee

Information is from the following websites: National Center for Educational Statistics; U.S. Bureau of the Census.

Questions about
Your School Crisis Plan

- Where is the crisis plan located?

- Do all teachers have a copy of the crisis plan in their classrooms?

- When was the crisis plan last revised?

- Which person or persons in this school are in charge during a schoolwide crisis?

- What types of crises are covered in your school's crisis plan?

- Are there any duties outlined specifically for you?

- During a lockdown, what are your responsibilities?

- What is the custodian responsible for during a lockdown?

- Does your school have a phone tree? If so, how does it work? Is the phone tree up-to-date?

- Does your school have a crisis team? If so, who participates on the crisis team?

- Does your crisis plan say anything about reporting suspected abuse?

- If a news reporter covers a school crisis, with whom should he or she talk?

- Does your school's crisis plan provide information about referring a student who is talking about suicide?

- Who helps with medical emergencies?

- Are there secret or confidential code words the principal uses to alert staff to the presence of an emergency over the intercom?

- Does the crisis plan include any information on natural disasters (e.g., flood, tornado, earthquake)?

Role Playing
Crisis Scenarios

Note: During crisis situations you typically do not have the luxury of time. The role plays in this exercise are designed to give you an opportunity to "think on your feet," problem solve, and experience the immediacy and intensity of feelings associated with crisis situations.

ROLE PLAY 1

You are the secretary for an elementary school. You are talking with a student (Tami) who was recently in an automobile accident (3 weeks ago). Although Tami suffered only minor injuries, the father and younger sister were seriously injured and died soon after the accident. The student is in the office crying. Role-play how you would respond to this situation.

Questions to consider:

- What information is missing from this scenario that would influence your response?
- How busy/noisy is the office area?
- What strategies could you use to calm this student?
- If the student settles down, stops crying, and goes back to class, would you still need to tell anyone about the student's visit to the office?
- What would you do if the student did not calm down and stop crying?
- Would you refer this student to the school's mental health professional (counselor, social worker, or school psychologist)?

ROLE PLAY 2

You are a teacher at the middle school. It is 3:00 (right after the junior high bell rings to release students). Three friends of a 14-year-old girl come into your classroom and tell you that they are concerned about Jessica because she told them that she "did not think life was worth living any more." Her friends say that Jessica has progressively become more withdrawn and depressed over the last month. As a teacher, what would you do?

Questions to consider:

- What advice should you, as the teacher, give to Jessica's friends?
- Does the school crisis plan tell teachers what to do when a student makes suicidal statements?
- Do you have a positive relationship with Jessica and her parent/guardian? Are parent/guardian emergency phone numbers available in the office?
- Can you contact the school's mental health professional and express concerns?
- What should you do if the student has already left the school?

Assignment: Review your school's crisis plan. List your responsibilities in helping with the following situations: school lockdown, helping a student who is upset and crying, responding to a student's suicidal comments, and reporting abuse.

CRISIS RESPONSE SKILLS

LEND A HELPING HAND

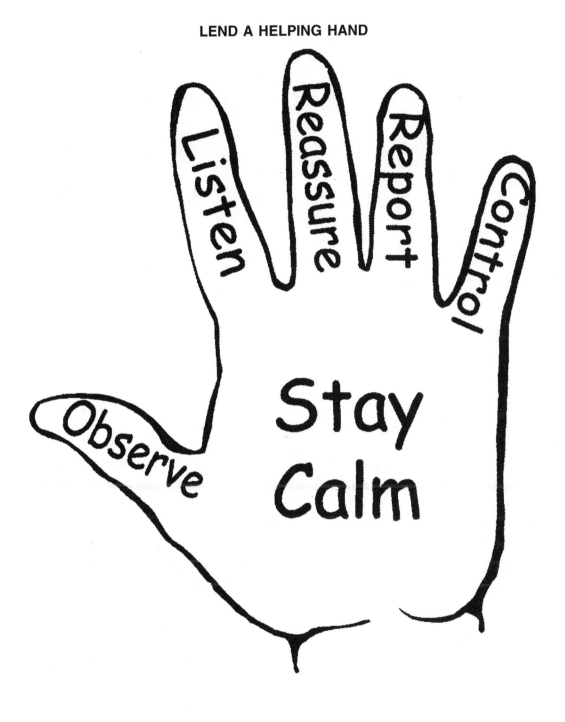

3

Communication

How to Listen, What to Say, and How to React

Melissa Allen Heath *and* Annette Jerome

BASIC SKILLS IN PROVIDING EMOTIONAL SUPPORT

Offering emotional first aid to students and adults consists of knowing how to communicate effectively, and most importantly, how to listen. Good communication skills are not limited to counselors or psychologists. These skills are used every day in supporting students.

A basic list of effective communication skills is reviewed in this chapter. Some of these skills are easy to describe and require little explanation. However, others are difficult to describe and require more explanation. Good communication skills provide the means to strengthen and support students in need of emotional first aid. (Note: If you are reviewing communication skills in a staff training, use Overhead 3.1, "Fundamentals of Good Listening Skills," at the end of the chapter.)

One of the most basic skills in listening is *empathy*. Empathy is often misunderstood. Some think empathy and sympathy are the same. However, *sympathy* means you are feeling sorry for the person; sympathy drains your emotional energy. Empathy gives you power—it means you are trying to understand the other person and how he or she is thinking and feeling. Empathy does not include feeling sorry for others. When you are assisting

Annette Jerome, PhD, School Psychologist, Hurst–Euless–Bedford Independent School District (Texas).

others in need, always remember that no matter how serious the situation, an individual has the power to rise above it and come out stronger for it. Children are incredibly resilient. Empathy will help the other person feel cared for and understood.

Show you care by listening intently, giving the student your total attention. Position yourself at eye level with him or her. Respond with understanding statements to reflect the student's statements. Reflective statements must fit your style, but examples include: "That must be tough" and "You must be going through a difficult time right now." Sometimes your care and concern are demonstrated more by *how* you say something than by the actual words you use.

Another attribute of good communications skills is *sincerity*. Being sincere in what you say and how you respond goes a long way in building trust. Students are extremely sensitive in detecting insincerity and phoniness. When an individual is genuine, a foundation of trust is built, supporting a healthy relationship.

Often when students are in crisis, they feel isolated and alone and are in need of *reassurance*. Reassure with statements such as "You are not alone" and "I am here for you." Students need to feel connected, particularly when they are dealing with personal problems. Some suggestions to decrease isolation and involve students in campus life include starting friendship groups for lunch, training students to assist in the counseling office, providing a mentoring program for students, utilizing student volunteers to help students who have special needs, providing a student support network so all students feel included in the school activities, and mixing groups of students on school planning committees to increase student support and interaction.

REFERRING TO A PROFESSIONAL

All staff and teachers need to be familiar with the guidelines for turning student problems over to the counselor or mental health professional. In cases where the student is a danger to him- or herself or is threatening someone else's safety, you must refer the case to a professional, even if the student tries to make you promise to keep it a secret. Also, students exhibiting extreme or unusual behaviors should be referred to the mental health professional.

STRENGTHENING COMMUNICATION SKILLS

If you want to strengthen your communication skills, there are also things you should avoid. Do not say, "I know just what you mean." No one ever totally understands another person's suffering. Each person is unique and deserves to be seen as an individual. However, it is appropriate to say, "I am trying to understand what you are experiencing."

Avoid "one-upping"—that is, telling a personal story that minimizes the student's experience by inference. In other words, your story of pain and suffering is more severe than the student's situation. It is best to limit your personal stories when assisting others. Others are more in need of a good listening ear, not a preachy sermon or a lot of details about things you have experienced.

Beware of inappropriate boundaries. Keep an appropriate emotional distance and avoid becoming overinvolved. Red flags warning of inappropriate boundaries include loss of composure, letting the student become overly dependent on you, letting the student call you at home to discuss emotional issues or family issues, and keeping secrets that should be reported to protect the student (e.g., suicidal comments, descriptions of abuse). Do *not* promise to keep a secret. The welfare and safety of students are more important than keeping a secret. Sometimes adults display inappropriate boundaries because of past personal experiences that have caused them great pain. They over-identify with the student's problems and lose their sense of balance. It is very important to set limits and to get professional help for students who require more extensive support.

LISTENING TO STUDENTS IN CRISIS: BASIC LISTENING SKILLS

Note: The following section can be formatted into an inservice presentation for teachers and staff. Handout 3.1 is provided at the end of the chapter as a summary of the information. Worksheets 3.1 and 3.2 are included to accompany this training.

Sometimes students share disappointments or concerns with teachers and staff. When students are upset and emotional, they may feel more comfortable talking to someone they know and trust. Although teachers and staff are not trained counselors, they can be good listeners. In preparing teachers and staff to be supportive of students, it is important to teach them the basics of good listening skills. The following overview of skills will assist them in providing better support to students.

Position

It is important to help students feel comfortable. Position yourself on eye level with students to convey the message that you are right there with them. Stay in close proximity but make sure you give them adequate personal space. Also, be sensitive to student diversity. Some students may avoid eye contact to show respect or deference to an authority figure or adult. In some situations, however, students may avoid eye contact because they are uncomfortable, fearful, or distrustful.

Although sitting may help to relax some students, others, particularly boys, may be more comfortable taking a short walk down the hall or on school grounds. Have a stress ball, special pens, or other small objects available so students have something to do with their hands. When active students keep their hands busy, it reduces nervous tension and helps them feel less self-conscious about talking.

Body Language

Good listening requires the adult to clear his or her mind of worries and concentrate on what the student is saying and doing. The listener must (1) be aware of his or her own facial expressions and posture, (2) remain calm, and (3) not overreact to the student's situation.

The adult must be aware of the student's body language, watching for gestures, signs of nervous energy, and contradictions between the student's words and behaviors. Watching for unspoken messages in body language is just as important as listening to the student's words.

A video clip from the movie *As Good as It Gets* provides a good example of how people overreact during crisis situations. The clip begins in the hospital room. Simon, the artist, is lying in the hospital bed, his face distorted, swollen, bruised, and crisscrossed with black stitches. His friend Jackie walks into the room, unaware of the seriousness of Simon's injuries. As she enters the room, she tries to be upbeat as she cheerfully greets him, saying, "How are you doing, great one?" She walks around the side of his bed, catching her first glimpse of his facial injuries. Breaking into sobs, she gasps for breath and reacts in horror to Simon's hideous face. Simon is watching her reaction carefully. His fear mounts. He tenuously admits, "I haven't looked at myself yet. I figured I could tell from your reaction. . . ." Frank, the art dealer, then enters the room. After seeing Simon's face, he halts his conversation, yelps in horror, and slumps into a chair.

Both Jackie's and Frank's reactions are extreme. This example demonstrates the importance of remaining calm when others need to be strengthened. The video clip ends with Simon asking Jackie for a mirror. Raising the mirror to his face, he slowly and tearfully takes his first look. Tears stream down Jackie's face as she watches for his reaction.

Using Video Clip to Demonstrate Body Language Skill

For inservice training, prior to showing the hospital scene from *As Good as It Gets*, give a brief synopsis of the movie's plot. Then give a few details to introduce the clip. Ask these questions before showing the clip:

- Do those in charge remain calm?
- How would you describe their facial expressions?

After showing the video clip, ask the group to evaluate Jackie's and Frank's body language. Discuss strategies for coping with situations that catch you off guard. How will you remain in control and prevent yourself from overreacting? Think of examples that would demonstrate the importance of remaining calm.

In times of extreme stress, teachers and staff must remain calm. Their support will be an anchor of stability for students. Situations quickly escalate when adults in charge do not control their emotions, particularly during times of crisis. Students look to the adults in their lives for a sense of security.

Speech

During a tense situation, whether a full-blown crisis or a difficult conversation with individual students, *how* the adult speaks is important. Although there are times when a raised voice is needed, a soft, calm voice is more likely to deescalate an emotional situation. Slow the rate of speech, making each word count. Remember the two-part "see-saw" rule (see Overhead 3.2 at the end of the chapter): The louder the student's voice, the softer your voice; the faster the student speaks, the slower you speak.

When students feel out of control, adults must remain in control. In times of crisis, personal or schoolwide, students search for an anchor. Adults must be confident and genuine. Words are important. Use caring statements that validate students' experiences, such as "That sounds tough" and "This must be a difficult time for you." Reassure students with statements such as "You are not alone" and "I am here for you."

Action Plan

It is important to direct students from the passive victim stage to the proactive stage. After talking with students, help them to take the next step by asking, "Where do we go from here?" If problems are extreme or if the situation requires professional attention, consult with the school's mental health professional. You might say: "We have talked about some really tough things. Let's talk more with the counselor about your concerns."

If professional support is not needed because problems involve normal adjustment issues, encourage students to talk with friends or other adults. Ask "Who can you talk to about your worries?" Always let them know they are not alone. Others can and will help.

Follow-Up

After talking with a student, it is important to let him or her know you will be there in the future for him or her. Agree upon a time and place for a check-in. You might say "Let's talk again tomorrow after class." If the student's problems are serious, the adult should talk with the school's mental health professional. The counselor will assist in determining if the student would benefit from counseling or if the parent should be notified. The mental health professionals in the school are trained to assist teachers and staff with difficult problems.

The video *Lean on Me* has a good example of an action plan and follow-up skills. A clip of Principal Joe Clark counseling an emotional student, Kanesha, in the school hallway shows how he moves her from a passive victim role to an active problem-solving role. This clip would be an effective supplement to training teachers and staff about good listening skills.

Background: *Lean on Me* is based on the true story of Joe Clark, the controversial African American principal of Eastside High School in New Jersey. Joe Clark was an advocate of tough-love education. Under his leadership the school rose out of violence, crime, drugs, and low achievement to become a strong academically oriented school. His motto was "If you don't succeed in life, I want you to blame yourselves."

This clip of Kanesha and the principal is an excellent demonstration of moving from information gathering to specifying an action plan and follow-up. Although the principal is tough talking and direct, he has a long history with the student and her family. Although he is not a perfect example of a caring and empathic person, he is effective in drawing Kanesha out of her shell and getting her to talk. He calls her by name. Reminding her of their previous connection, he says, "I've known you more than half your life." He also points out a personal strength, telling her that she is a smart girl.

Within a few sentences he gets to the heart of the matter: Kanesha is at risk for foster home placement. The student trusts the principal because he knows her and her family. As Kanesha cries, he becomes directive and starts to problem solve. He takes Kanesha's arm and says "Come with me. Come on. I'll see what I can do about this." He walks with Kanesha directly to the counselor. In the student's presence, Mr. Clark asks the counselor to pull the student's file and talk with her. He then says: "Get back to me."

Following this scene the principal and counselor go to visit Kanesha's home. The mother knows the principal, who has been part of the community for many years. Although the movie shows a great deal of controversy surrounding the principal, he wants what is best for students. Kanesha and her mother feel supported by the principal. He is effective in helping the student through this crisis.

When the school has a long and positive history with families, school staff can be highly effective in helping students with problems. There is no substitute for time in forming a relationship. Daily contact with students helps form strong relationships and builds a broader base of support. With this support, students feel comfortable sharing problems with teachers and staff who have their best interests at heart. Daily contact is also conducive to making action plans and following up with students.

TEACHING LISTENING SKILLS

Short video clips provide an inexpensive, effective, and entertaining way to teach critical communication skills. Listed below are descriptions of several video clips containing brief conversations that demonstrate listening skills. The exaggerated nature of the interactions makes it easier to observe and critique listening skills (or their lack) in each scenario. Prior to watching the video clips, review Handout 3.1, "Listening to Students in Crisis: Basic Listening Skills." This handout lists five basic elements of good listening skills. In addition to watching video clips, role-playing and discussing the skills can augment the learning process.

The success of using video clips hinges on the organizational skills of the presenter. Cue each video clip before the inservice training. Table 3.1 indicates starting and stopping points for the video clips. Prior to showing the clip, give a brief story line as background. To assist in focusing attention, review the main points of information immediately before showing the clip. Present the clip, then briefly discuss the main points. To assist participants in evaluating listening skills portrayed in each video clip, Worksheets 3.1 and 3.2 are provided. These worksheets include a checklist to assist participants in reviewing critical aspects of effective listening and also help structure discussion following the video clip.

TABLE 3.1. Cueing Video Clips for Listening Skills

Video (length of clip)	Clip description	Start	End
As Good as It Gets (60 seconds)	Hospital bed scene; Simon with facial scars. Clip starts 20 minutes into the movie; for DVD, 24 seconds into frame 6/28.	Jackie enters the hospital room. Simon is in bed. Start the clip right before Jackie says, "How are you doing, great one?"	After Jackie and Frank overreact to Simon's scarred face, Simon looks into Jackie's hand mirror. End the clip right after Jackie hands Simon the mirror.
Lean on Me (70 seconds)	Principal and Kanesha sitting on couch in school hall. Clip starts 45 minutes into the movie.	After fighting in the hall with a drug dealer, the principal comes back to his office. Kanesha is sitting on a couch outside the office door. As he looks down the hall toward Kanesha, he shuts the office door. Start the clip just prior to their conversation.	The principal tells the counselor what needs to be done for Kanesha. Stop the clip right after the counselor says: "Come on, Kanesha."
City Slickers (105 seconds)	Tent scene with Mitch and Phil. Clip starts 78 minutes into the movie; for DVD, 3 minutes 45 seconds into frame 14/16.	After Phil held the gun to the bully's head, he walks into the tent. Cue the film on Mitch kneeling in front of Phil in the tent.	After Phil says: "I'm alone . . . ," two men come to the door of the tent and interrupt the conversation. Stop the video when Phil and Mitch's conversation is interrupted.
A Christmas Story (125 seconds)	Ralphie on Santa's lap. Clip starts 68 minutes into the movie; for DVD, on frame 24/32.	Ralphie is standing in line to talk with Santa. Start the clip when it is Ralphie's turn to sit on Santa's lap.	After Ralphie says what he *really* wants for Christmas, he is shoved down the slide. Stop when he arrives at the bottom of the slide.
As Good as It Gets (95 seconds)	Middle-of-the-night Chinese soup. Clip starts 56 minutes into the movie; for DVD 30 seconds into frame 16/28.	Melvin brings Chinese soup to Simon in the middle of the night. Melvin knocks on Simon's door. Start the clip with Simon opening his door.	Melvin says, "I'm glad we did this. Good talking to you." Melvin stands up and walks out the door. Stop the clip when Simon is sitting alone on the bench.

Video Clip: *City Slickers*

In *City Slickers*, three friends go on a vacation herding cattle in New Mexico to escape their troubled lives. Hot weather, harsh conditions, and mean-spirited bullies push the group to the edge of sanity. The video clip from *City Slickers* demonstrates both good and bad examples of listening skills. In particular, this clip does *not* contain two important messages a person in crisis needs to hear:

1. It is important to acknowledge how difficult things feel to a person in crisis. Never downplay feelings by saying "It's not that bad." Validation of feelings is key in demonstrating empathy. A good listener might say: "That sounds really tough" or "Things must be really hard for you right now."

2. Another important message a good listener communicates to the person in crisis is "You are not alone. I am here for you." Often someone who is experiencing difficulties feels isolated and alone. He or she may feel that no one cares. To counter these feelings, the listener must communicate "I am here for you and I care about you." It is important for the individual to feel supported.

In this video clip, everyone is exhausted. Those in charge of leading the cattle drive are overbearing, and they harass the inexperienced vacationers. Phil, typically meek and mild mannered, threatens the bullies and in a fit of anger holds a gun to one bully's head. Immediately after subduing the bullies, Phil retreats into the tent with his gun. He sits down. His two friends, Ed and Mitch, follow him. They are worried about Phil. He seems on the edge of an emotional breakdown.

Cue the film to this point. Start the clip with Mitch (Billy Crystal) kneeling down directly in front of Phil. This is a very powerful conversation. First Phil says he is OK, then as Mitch listens, Phil confides in his friend. Phil describes his life as a total mess. He stares at the gun as he talks and begins to cry. Mitch tries to comfort Phil. Phil breaks down, giving details about why his life is so horrible. Mitch tells Phil "It's not that bad." At the close of the conversation Phil says "I'm all alone." This phrase hangs in silence with no supportive comment from Mitch. Their talk is interrupted when two men come to the door of the tent. End the clip.

The *City Slickers* clip is already evaluated on Worksheet 3.1. After showing the clip, review comments on the worksheet to demonstrate how to evaluate the remaining video clips. Discuss both positive and negative points regarding the listening skills. What worked well? What did not? Discuss the two weak points: when Mitch said "It's not that bad" and when Mitch did not respond to Phil's statement "I'm all alone."

Video Clip: *A Christmas Story*

This is a movie about 9-year-old Ralphie, whose life is totally absorbed with the goal of obtaining a Genuine Red Ryder Carbine Action 200-Shot Lightning Loader Range Model Air Rifle (Red Ryder BB Gun). Safety-minded grownups, including his parents, constantly remind Ralphie that this gun is not safe. His frustration builds as he repeatedly hears the phrase "You'll shoot your eye out." After his request is refused time and again by his parents, Ralphie's last hope is to ask Santa.

The video clip starts with Ralphie and his little brother standing in a long line of children, eagerly waiting to tell Santa what they want for Christmas. It is 9:00 on Christmas Eve, and the store is closing. Elves yank children forward to move the line along faster. They yell orders for children to "get moving" and to quit dragging their feet. Terrified children scream in fear. Finally it is Ralphie's turn. He is pulled up the stairs by an impatient elf and plunked on Santa's lap. The scene is tense. Ask these questions prior to showing the video clip *A Christmas Story*.

- How do Santa and the elves listen to Ralphie?
- What is Santa's agenda?
- When Ralphie is finally able to tell Santa what he really wants for Christmas, how does Santa respond?

Show the clip. Ask participants to complete the column under *A Christmas Story* on Worksheet 3.2.

Summary of video clip: This is Ralphie's last hope of ever getting the Red Ryder BB gun. The elves are pressuring Ralphie to hurry. Santa bellows "Ho Ho Ho" repeatedly. Again the elves exhort: "Hurry, the store is closing. We have a lot of people waiting." Overwhelmed, Ralphie forgets what he wants for Christmas. Disoriented, Ralphie agrees with Santa's suggestion, a football. Ralphie is ousted from Santa's lap and shoved down the slide. With all the effort he can muster, Ralphie yells "No" and frantically pulls himself up the slide toward Santa. He blurts out that he wants the Red Ryder BB gun. To Ralphie's fervent and hopeful request, Santa matter-of-factly states the dreaded words: "You'll shoot your eye out. Merry Christmas. Ho Ho Ho." Santa shoves his boot in Ralphie's face. Ralphie screams "No" all the way down the slide. At the bottom of the slide he lies defeated in the fake snow.

Evaluate Santa and Ralphie's interaction in terms of the five listening skills on Worksheet 3.2. Discuss participants' responses.

1. *Position*: Although Santa and Ralphie were initially on eye-to-eye level, Ralphie was uncomfortable. There was not enough personal space—Santa's face was right in Ralphie's face.
2. *Body language*: Santa did not clear his mind and concentrate on the child. He was impatient, and he rushed Ralphie. Santa had one thing on his mind: getting done. He did not pay attention to Ralphie's body language. Ralphie was tense and could not remember what he wanted to say. Rather than giving Ralphie more time to speak, Santa rushed Ralphie and even supplied Ralphie's Christmas request: "football."
3. *Speech*: Santa's speech was rushed and loud: "Ho Ho Ho." Santa did not use caring statements to show empathy for Ralphie's nervousness or his intensity about the Red Ryder BB gun. Santa's language demonstrated an "I don't care" attitude.
4. *Action plan*: Santa had no action plan for Ralphie. Santa had one thing on his mind: to get through the line of children quickly and finish his job for the night. Santa did not assist with problem-solving strategies.
5. *Follow-up*: Santa did not have a follow-up plan. He did not let Ralphie know that he would be there for him in the future.

Video Clip: *As Good as It Gets*

This movie clip provides a good example of the hopeless and exhausting feeling of living with depression. It also provides an example of poor listening skills. Provide a brief background of the scene prior to showing the video clip.

Background: It is 3:22 in the morning. Melvin puts on his slippers and goes across the hall of the apartment building to take his neighbor (Simon) some Chinese soup. Simon is depressed and homebound, convalescing from serious injuries. These injuries were sustained a few weeks earlier when he was brutally attacked in his home by burglars. His medical bills have depleted his bank account. He feels he has nothing to live for. Observe how these two men do not talk to each other—they talk *at* each other. More accurately, they talk to themselves; they have a parallel conversation.

Start the video clip with Simon opening the door. Notice how Melvin positions himself in relation to Simon. More specifically, watch for eye contact and body language. Listen carefully to Melvin's comments. Does he make caring, reassuring, supportive statements to validate and show understanding of Simon's difficult situation? Watch carefully for any caring statements that might reflect the pain Simon is feeling. Note how their conversation ends. The video clip ends with Melvin walking out and Simon sitting alone on the bench.

After viewing the clip, use Worksheet 3.2 to make notes and provide structure for discussing the following points:

1. *Position*: Melvin came in and sat on the bench with Simon, placing the Chinese soup between them. Although they were on the same level, Melvin faced forward and did not engage in eye contact with Simon.
2. *Body language*: Melvin was weighed down with his own worries, aware only of his own feelings. He ignored Simon's obviously uncomfortable body language. Simon hobbled to the bench, apparently in physical pain. Simon struggled to express his thoughts. He had a hopeless look on his face as he spoke, and his posture was slumped.
3. *Speech*: Melvin spoke slowly and quietly. He sighed and focused on his own depression. He did not offer any caring statements to support Simon or acknowledge Simon's physical and emotional pain.
4. *Action plan*: Melvin gets up to leave right after Simon says, "You can barely find the will to complain." In parting, Melvin states, "I'm glad we did this. Good talking to you." Melvin gave no guidance or hope for future direction. As the scene ends, Simon looks puzzled, alone on the bench.
5. *Follow-up*: Melvin gave no indication he planned to check on Simon in the future.

SUMMARY OF GOOD LISTENING SKILLS

In summary, good listening is broken down into five areas of basic skills: position, body language, speech, action plan, and follow-up. It is important to think about how you communicate with students and, in particular, how you listen when students talk to you about difficult situations in their lives.

Discuss these questions:

- Which of these skills come naturally to you when you are listening to students?
- Which listening skills are more difficult for you and will require some practice?
- Using Handout 3.1, review the skills. On a separate sheet of paper, evaluate your listening skills in each area.

COMMUNICATING WITH COMMUNITY MENTAL HEALTH PROFESSIONALS

In some situations, crisis intervention services may need to expand beyond the typical counseling services provided by school professionals. In considering outside referrals, schools must become more familiar with community resources, particularly those resources dedicated to serving minority groups and non-English-speaking populations. Alternative services may include community support groups, religious leaders aligned with the family's belief system, shelters for the homeless, protective shelters for battered women and children, free or reduced mental health services, clinics serving medical and dental needs, Red Cross services, community transportation services, and so on.

Many schools employ social workers to assist with these varied needs. However, administrators, school psychologists, and school counselors can also assist families in accessing services. Most communities publish a book of local resources and services provided through the United Way. Additionally, emergency numbers, such as an abuse hotline, suicide hotline, and runaway hotline, are listed in the front of the phone book.

As school personnel interface with personnel in community services, relationships are formed. An understanding between the school and agency leaders develops, further easing access to services for students and families. Selecting a single contact person from the school is helpful in forming a relationship with community agencies. It is suggested that teachers and staff refer their concerns to this point person. The principal should be informed of referrals and reasons for those referrals. Keeping records of referrals and phone calls to agencies is highly recommended. Worksheet 3.3, "Emergency Contact Log," is provided at the end of the chapter to assist practitioners in documenting community referrals and phone calls for emergency situations. For instance, in cases of reporting suspected abuse, this form can document calls to Child Protective Services. (Additional information about child abuse is contained in Chapter 5.)

It is important to follow your school district's policy for documenting emergency calls. Some districts require school employees to submit a short written report documenting calls made to Child Protective Services. These records may be kept in a central district office location, such as with the district's Special Services Coordinator. Some districts have a policy for keeping emergency contact records with the school nurse or school counselor. Keeping accurate records provides a way to track incidents of abuse across time.

Reporting Suspected Abuse

By law, all adults are required to report suspected abuse to Child Protective Services or the Department of Human Services. You do not have to prove there has been abuse, only that you suspect abuse. Calls of suspected abuse are either reported to a local office's number or to a toll-free 800 number. The 800 number is operational 24 hours a day, 7 days a week; however, there may be a long wait before you talk with someone. Helpful information to give the authorities includes name of student, age, address, home phone, what type of abuse you suspect, and the reason for your suspicion. Give facts: "This is what I saw. . . ." "This is what was said. . . ." "This is why I am reporting this case of suspected abuse. . . ." Never pry information from the student you suspect is being abused. Do not ask additional questions to clarify the student's story. Let the student vent his or her feelings, but leave the fact finding to the proper authorities.

School personnel are on the front line of identifying needs and accessing services for students in need of emotional support and guidance. Particularly during times of crisis, great care must be taken in responding effectively and with sensitivity to students' needs. Teachers and staff need clear guidelines for when and how to refer a student to other professionals. Questions should be initially directed to the school's mental health professional (school counselor, social worker, or school psychologist), who is more experienced in determining the student's needs and how best to meet those needs.

COMMUNICATING WITH PARENTS

Schools must communicate with parents, particularly after a crisis or traumatic event. Parents need to be informed about how the school is handling stressful situations and what services are offered to assist students. Parents and the school should develop a comfortable partnership in assisting the student. Parents should be on equal footing with the school in communicating information; however, parents always have the major control over which interventions will ultimately be used with their children.

All students are affected by both personal and schoolwide problems. However, each student is individual in how he or she reacts to, or copes with, trauma. Sometimes parents do not recognize their own child's reactions to trauma. Furthermore, they may have a tendency to deny that there is a problem. Informing parents of problems at school, whether emotional, behavioral, or academic in nature, is always a difficult task. The manner in which a parent is informed can set the stage and the tenor for future interactions. Great care should be taken in conveying the news that there is a problem or suggestions for how to "fix" the problem.

Parents must be treated with respect. School personnel must always acknowledge parents' contribution to student success during good times, so that when negative news must be shared there is a previous history of positive communication in place to act as a buffer. Relationships become strained when judgmental statements are made or inferred. It is best to remain positive and nonjudgmental.

Parents may be unaware of how children react to trauma and not know what to do, or how to help their child. It is important to share basic information without overdoing it. A one-page handout highlighting basic information is preferable to a stack of academic articles or books on the topic. Parents lead busy lives and need things simplified to avoid feeling overwhelmed.

It is helpful for parents to know what is considered normal. Children commonly react to trauma by reverting (regressing) to immature behaviors. For instance, children may want to climb in bed with the parent after a nightmare. Bedwetting, thumbsucking, and clinginess may overwhelm parents, unless they realize that these are normal responses to trauma for a child of a certain age. In addition, parents should be encouraged to maintain family routines during stressful times.

In order to gauge the severity of a child's response to stress or trauma, parents should be aware of changes in the child's sleeping, eating, and behavior patterns. Children may exhibit extreme behavior changes, particularly in expressing anger or sadness. It is important for parents to limit media exposure to traumatic events. Witnessing an event over and over on television can make the event even more traumatic to the child or adolescent.

Ideally, parents/guardians know their child better than anyone else. They have insights about how their child copes with stress. Consulting with parents and forming a partnership allows interventions to be consistent across settings. Helping parents locate a variety of available resources is essential. However, when offering suggestions, it is important to be sensitive to their preferences in seeking help.

COMMUNICATING WITH THE MEDIA

Most school districts have a designated spokesperson who is responsible for communicating with the media and making official statements for the district. During a crisis, this individual works closely with the local news stations and newspaper offices. The spokesperson's statements are scrutinized by the superintendent and approved for release.

It is important for a school district to have a positive relationship with the media. School districts and the media need to come to an understanding about how to handle certain topics. For instance, when the media is covering an incident involving a student suicide, placing the story on the front page or giving this topic high priority is detrimental to both the community and the school district. The American Foundation for Suicide Prevention has website information geared specifically for the media. The information includes tips for writing responsible and appropriate news reports on suicides.

Building a good relationship with the media includes setting expectations for future interactions. For instance, when an event is covered on campus, many times reporters are eager to solicit comments from students and teachers. The principal and spokesperson for the district should discuss ahead of time how these events will be covered most effectively without compromising student safety and well-being.

Teachers and staff must resist the urge to make comments to the media regarding school incidents, crises, or controversial topics. The district spokesperson or principal should provide school employees with a set of guidelines for interacting with the media.

However, during a crisis, responding with "no comment" may be just as harmful as making a comment. "No comment" suggests an uncaring attitude or makes it appear that there is something to cover up or hide. An example of saying something other than "no comment" might include the following comments: "This is a very painful time for our school. I am saddened by this event." If you are pressured by the media to give information, you might say "I don't know the facts right now, but when information is available, the school spokesperson will provide the facts."

SUGGESTED READING

Brooks, B., & Siegel, P. M. (1996). *The scared child: Helping kids overcome traumatic events*. New York: Wiley.

Fearn-Banks, K. (2002). *Crisis communications: A casebook approach* (2nd ed.). Mahwah, NJ: Erlbaum.

Jerome, A., & Mukamal, A. (2005). *Parent training and support program and materials: MEMOS for Parents*—activities to help parents communicate with children and provide positive behavior supports. Available for purchase: $50. Contact information: *annette.jerome@att.net* or call 940-594-8487.

U.S. Department of Health and Human Services. (2002). *Communication in a crisis: Risk communication guidelines for public officials*. Washington, DC: Author.

WEBSITES

www.afsp.org/education/recommendations/index.htm

Reporting on suicide: Recommendations for the media. Sponsored by the American Foundation for Suicide Prevention.

www.thirteen.org/edonline/concept2class/familycommunity/index_sub1.html

From the workshop: *Making Family and Community Connections*. Sponsored by the Educational Broadcasting Corporation (2004).

Listening Skills (Part 1)

Review Handout 3.1, "Listening to Students in Crisis." After watching each video clip, evaluate the listening skills of the adult in charge of the crisis situation. As an example, the evaluation of the first video is already completed.

City Slickers
(Tent Scene with Mitch and Phil)

(1) *Position*	GOOD: Close proximity: Mitch kneels down in front of Phil. Mitch uses good eye contact. It feels like he is right there with Phil.
(2) *Body Language*	GOOD: Mitch uses caring facial expressions. He focuses on Phil. Even though Phil says that everything is OK, Mitch sees that Phil is upset. Mitch is calm and does not overreact to the gun or Phil's emotional outburst.
(3) *Speech*	GOOD: Mitch talks softly, slowly, and calmly. He stays in control, even when Phil is out of control. Mitch uses a metaphor: "do-over." BAD: (1) Mitch says "It's not that bad." (2) When Phil says he is all alone, Mitch does **not** respond with support statements such as "I am here for you. You are not alone."
(4) *Action Plan*	Although not put in terms of realistic goals, the metaphor of the "do-over" gives hope for a future plan. It is an attempt to point Phil toward the future rather than having him dwell on the past.
(5) *Follow-Up*	They are interrupted, and no follow-up is mentioned.

Listening Skills (Part 2)

Watch each video clip and evaluate the listening skills of the adult in charge of the crisis situation.

	A Christmas Story (Santa Claus and Ralphie)	*As Good as It Gets* (Middle-of-the-night Chinese soup)
(1) *Position*		
(2) *Body Language*		
(3) *Speech*		
(4) *Action Plan*		
(5) *Follow-Up*		

Emergency Contact Log

Date	Student	Concern	Guardian and Phone #	Agency Contact and Phone #	Follow-Up Date — Comments

Listening to Students in Crisis: Basic Listening Skills

When students are upset and emotional, they feel more comfortable talking to someone they know and trust. Although teachers and staff are not trained counselors, they can support to students in crisis.

Position

Help students feel comfortable by positioning yourself on their eye level. This position says "I am here with you." Stay in close proximity but give them adequate personal space. Also, be sensitive to student diversity. Some students avoid eye contact to show respect to an authority figure. However, students may avoid eye contact because they are uncomfortable, fearful, or distrustful.

Some students are more relaxed sitting, whereas others, particularly boys, are more comfortable walking. Have a stress ball, special pens, or other small objects for students to fiddle with to keep their hands busy. This simple provision reduces nervous tension and helps students feel more comfortable talking.

Body Language

Good listening requires a clear mind. Put your own worries aside. Concentrate on what the student is saying and doing. Be aware of your own facial expressions and posture. Remain calm. Do not overreact to the situation.

Be aware of the student's body language, watching for gestures, signs of nervous energy, and contradictions between the student's words and behaviors. Watch for unspoken messages in body language.

In times of extreme stress, you must remain calm. Your calming support will be an anchor of stability for students.

Speech

During a tense situation, *how* you speak is important. A soft, calm voice can deescalate an emotional situation. Slow your rate of speech, making each word count. Remember the "see-saw" rule; the louder the student's voice, the softer your voice; the faster the student speaks, the slower you speak.

Be confident and genuine. Words are important. Use caring statements that validate students' experiences: *"That sounds tough." "This must be a difficult time for you."* Reassure students: *"You are not alone." "I am here for you."*

Action Plan

Direct students from the passive victim stage to the proactive stage. Help them to take the next step by asking *"Where do we go from here?"* If problems are extreme or if the situation requires professional attention, consult with the school's mental health professional. *"We have talked about some really tough things. Let's talk more with the counselor about your concerns."*

If problems involve normal adjustment issues, encourage students to talk with friends or other adults. Ask *"Who can you talk to about your worries?"* Always let them know they are not alone. Others can and will help.

Follow-Up

After talking with a student, let the student know you will continue to be there for him or her. Agree upon a time and place for a check-in. You might say: *"Let's talk again tomorrow after class."* If the student's problems are serious, talk with the school's mental health professional. The counselor will assist in determining if the student would benefit from counseling or if the parent should be notified.

There is no substitute for time in forming a relationship. Daily contact with students builds strong relationships and a broader base of support. Daily contact is conducive to making action plans and following up with students.

FUNDAMENTALS OF GOOD LISTENING

GOAL: INCREASE CARING SUPPORT FOR STUDENTS

Skill	What it looks/sounds like
Caring	Listen more than you talk. Reflect to show you understand: "That must be tough."
Being Real	Be genuine. Be yourself. Don't be fake.
Reassuring	"You are not alone." "I am here for you." "We are here to help."
Knowing Limits	Get professional advice for serious situations: • Suicidal comments • Danger to self or others • Illegal activities • Threat to school safety

It is also important to know what you should **not** do:

- Do **not** promise to keep a secret.
- Do **not** say: "I know just what you mean." No one ever totally understands another person.
- Do **not** get overinvolved. Maintain healthy boundaries.

STAY CALM

Pay attention to:
Rate of speech
Volume of speech

REMEMBER THE SEE-SAW EFFECT:

The louder the
student's voice

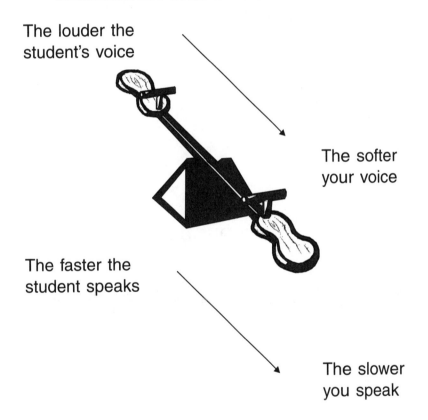

The softer
your voice

The faster the
student speaks

The slower
you speak

4

Children's Literature

A Resource to Assist with Crisis Intervention

DAWN SHEEN, MELISSA ALLEN HEATH, NATHAN JONES, EMILY HEATON,
and APRIL GSTETTENBAUER

INTRODUCTION

In an educational setting, bibliotherapy is a useful way for teachers to help students cope with daily challenges. Students need support to face the many challenges and problems confronting them today. They also need a foundation of hope to face the uncertainties ahead. Cognitive, affective, and/or behavioral functioning are affected as students try to make sense of difficult situations. The teacher can be influential in the healing process as he or she assists in providing support and hope. Although it is not appropriate for the teacher to offer professional counseling, steps can be taken in the classroom to help students understand and deal more effectively with challenging or stressful situations. Teachers can address specific issues by sharing children's literature and thereby positively impact their students.

Certain events affect the emotional functioning of many students at the same time (e.g., 9/11, a publicized kidnapping, the death of a classmate, natural disasters). On a

Nathan Jones, MS, School Psychologist, Campbell, California.
Emily Heaton, BS, Graduate Student in School Psychology, Brigham Young University, Provo, Utah.
April Gstettenbauer, BS, Ventura, California.

smaller scale, many students have difficulties maintaining relationships with friends and may fall into patterns of bullying, threatening, and endangering others. Students also carry burdens related to family life. Domestic violence, child abuse, and neglect pervade the homes of many innocent children. Students suffering the emotional aftereffects of violence and abuse often have difficulties focusing their attention on school-related work.

Based on Maslow's (1970) hierarchy of needs, when basic needs are not met, higher functioning, including the motivation to learn, is not realized. Many students worry about family finances, wondering if they will have food to eat or money to pay for daily living expenses. In some cases, families become transient or homeless. For these students, basic survival becomes their primary concern.

As they face daily challenges and cope with personal and societal problems, students struggle with ways of appropriately identifying and expressing their emotions. In a classroom setting, teachers have opportunities to model emotional processing, problem solving, and adaptive skills, either directly or with the help of resources such as children's literature. Effectively using children's literature helps students learn life skills and heal emotional wounds. In this chapter, the process of bibliotherapy is presented along with strategies to create a positive learning experience that leads to increased insight. Common distress signals indicating the need for outside intervention are also examined. A sample lesson plan utilizing bibliotherapy as well as tools to aid the teacher in selecting and keeping track of useful books are provided.

WHAT IS BIBLIOTHERAPY?

Sharing books or stories in order to help the reader or audience gain insight into personal problems or heal emotional wounds is called *bibliotherapy* (Doll & Doll, 1997; Pardeck & Pardeck, 1997). Appropriately sharing stories also creates a "safe distance" for students to deal with sensitive issues too difficult to face directly. Additionally, literature serves as a catalyst for healthy expression of emotion and developmental growth. Bibliotherapy is a means through which students learn to relate to a character with similar problems and draw conclusions about their own struggles. Stories provide alternative solutions to problems.

Although recognized as an effective therapeutic tool in counseling settings, bibliotherapy also has value in the school. For instance, schools directly emphasize the importance of literacy. By encouraging reading to promote personal development and healing, teachers achieve an educational goal while helping students gain personal insight and growth.

Bibliotherapy is helpful in addressing a variety of issues, ranging from developmental difficulties to severe emotional struggles (Pardeck, 1991). Pardeck (1995) states that "[bibliotherapy] is an innovative approach that teachers can use to help children deal with [their] problems" (p. 83). In a classroom setting, stories can assist students in gaining life skills and resolving developmental conflicts. Storytelling is also effective in meeting students' emotional needs in general crisis situations. Of course, the training and ability of the storyteller must be sufficient to address the specific issue.

STAGES OF BIBLIOTHERAPY

As the teacher appropriately uses literature to encourage growth and understanding, students progress through an internal process involving several stages (Nickerson, 1975). The first step is *involvement.* As the teacher shares the story, students listen and demonstrate interest in what is happening. Then, as they get "caught up" in the narrative, students begin to relate with characters in the book. This is called *identification.* Students best identify with characters that are similar in age and circumstance to themselves. In the third stage, *catharsis,* the characters deal with the situation in the story and students empathize with, and vicariously experience, the characters' feelings. When resolution to the characters' dilemma is found, students also release some emotional tension.

After releasing emotional tension, students move into the next stage, *insight.* Students begin to think about what happened in the story and apply it in their own lives. Problems that may have seemed insurmountable become less overwhelming as they see how someone in similar circumstances solved them. It is during this stage that students begin resolving the struggles they may be experiencing personally. *Universalization* (Ford, 2000) is the final stage during which students recognize that they are not alone in their problems. A sense of connection replaces isolation as students realize that others have similar struggles.

LITERATURE SELECTION

To draw students into the process, the story must be relevant to their lives, address the issue at hand, and be developmentally appropriate. Teachers need to demonstrate sensitivity to children's emotional capacity. When story issues are too intense, students feel overwhelmed and growth is impeded. An awareness of students' life situations and personalities is essential.

It is imperative to choose literature that meets the goals of bibliotherapy. Basically, a good story is honest and sensitive to religious and cultural beliefs. A good story also strengthens coping skills and provides support and hope (Allen, Stott, Jones, Heaton, & Gstettenbauer, 2003). Other characteristics of a good story include the following:

- Age-appropriate plot
- Realistic plot (not necessarily "happily ever after" ending; McIntyre, 1999)
- Resolution to a problem in which main character gains insight
- Multidimensional characters, not stereotyped (Tu, 1999)
- Accurate information

- Sensitive and accurate portrayal of individuals with disabilities
- A positive focus on what characters *can* do

It is also important to know which books should be avoided. Do not select stories with simplistic "Band-Aid" solutions, overdone and manipulative emotional scenes, overwhelming situations with little or no resolution, characters portrayed as victims *or* superheroes, inappropriate role models, or questionable standards or values not supported by the community.

TEACHING PROCESS

After choosing the book, the teacher decides how the story will be shared. Forgan (2002) discusses effective teaching strategies associated with bibliotherapy. Initial preparation involves building an appropriate foundation for the story by conducting prereading activities, such as discussing what students already know about the given topic. The teacher could begin by showing the picture on the cover, introducing the characters in the book, and asking students to imagine what will happen in the story. After preparing the students, guided reading begins.

During guided reading, the teacher reads the story aloud. Allen, Sheen, et al. (2003) provide suggestions for storytelling.

> Utilizing good story-telling techniques is essential to drawing students into the book. Familiarity with the story facilitates a natural and flowing presentation. Tone of voice brings the story and characters' feelings to life. Volume and rate of speech build the story's emotional intensity. Natural facial expressions and simple gestures model appropriate reaction and engage students' interest. Eye contact assists in assessing students' understanding and emotional reaction. Appropriate questions posed at the right time facilitate students' involvement and understanding. Providing a related activity following the story builds on the message and increases students' learning. (p. 13)

At the story's conclusion, students need time for reflection and closure as they absorb the situation in the book. Postreading activities that encourage growth and learning can provide the needed reflection and closure. During postreading, the teacher assesses how well the students understood the story. Having them retell the plot and discuss the characters' emotions are effective ways to measure comprehension. Another goal is to help students experience each stage of the bibliotherapy process. During a postreading discussion, "The students are asked probing questions, which helps them think about their feelings and better identify with the characters and events in the story" (McCarty & Chalmers, 1997, p. 12). The questions should require students to think on several different levels, from comprehension to analysis and synthesis.

Additionally, the teacher can enhance student learning with the use of experiential activities (Pardeck, 1995). The effects of bibliotherapy are strengthened as students participate in creative activities such as developing games, drawing, group processing, collaborating on a group story, writing alternative endings, journaling, or setting goals. Also useful are role plays, skits, or dramatic readings of the story. When preparing postreading activities, ask yourself: "What will best assist the students in connecting with the story and making conclusions that give the story personal meaning and relevance?"

Collaboration with parents and other professionals increases awareness of individual student needs. It is beneficial to seek parental support when addressing sensitive topics. Additionally, parents should be advised when their child's behavior is more extreme than expected. Consultation with the school's mental health professional is essential when students overreact emotionally or behaviorally. Counselors and school psychologists have the training necessary to assist with the healing process when the issue at hand requires more individualized attention.

SIGNS OF DISTRESS

In order to determine if students need extra help, the teacher should be aware of their reactions to the story. Good literature is a powerful tool that may elicit overwhelmingly strong feelings. Sometimes it is difficult for students to effectively process emotions, and their behavior may become disruptive. A change in a student's disposition or behavior patterns may indicate emotional distress. During reading, the teacher may observe restlessness, fearfulness, or behaviors typical of younger children. Students also may vocally express emotion or complain of physical illness. Being knowledgeable about developmentally appropriate behaviors is vital.

Children are often fidgety. The teacher may observe restlessness when the book is too long or the physical environment is uncomfortable. However, when a student is restless only during emotionally intense parts of the story, additional intervention is required. Constant, disruptive movement may also indicate inner turmoil. In emotional situations, students may temporarily regress to younger behaviors to comfort themselves. Persistent or recurring regressive behavior may indicate that the student lacks the ability to resolve emotional pain. In such cases the teacher should seek additional help from parents and the school counselor.

It is normal for students to empathize with a character that is in danger; however, excessive fearfulness is a sign of more serious distress. The ability of students to distinguish between actual and fictional danger is an important consideration when selecting stories. Occasionally, students respond to a story with extreme fear. Consultation with others is recommended when a student's fear is out of proportion to the actual danger presented in the story.

Effective use of bibliotherapy may elicit strong vocal responses. Students may want to interrupt the story with questions and comments. They may want to process their feelings immediately. In a group setting, this behavior may be disruptive and interfere with others' participation. Encouraging appropriate expression of emotion is an important part of the therapeutic process. However, when uncontrollable emotional outbursts occur, it is indicative of deeper distress. If students refuse to be comforted by the teacher or their peers, intervention outside the classroom is needed. The teacher should contact the parents and the school counselor for assistance.

Finally, students may complain of physical problems. When a student internalizes overwhelming emotion, the body may react with physical pain. Paying attention to the severity and frequency of the complaints is essential to determining the level of distress. When students indicate physical pain only during emotionally charged scenes, it may indicate that they are unable to recognize and express feelings. The teacher should be sensitive to these calls for help and respond with individualized attention and a referral to the school counselor.

In summary, students respond to stories in a variety of ways. The teacher must be aware of when students' behavior indicates distress. Tuning in to precursors of troubled behavior and monitoring the frequency and duration of such behavior are essential skills that distinguish mere storytelling from bibliotherapy. More serious intervention may be needed if:

- Students act out *only* during emotional parts of the story
- The reaction is more intense than anticipated
- The behavior lasts longer than expected

SUMMARY

Knowing the students, their personalities, and their situations will assist the teacher in selecting literature appropriate to facilitate growth. Children's literature is particularly useful in a school setting to help students cope with difficult situations. Stories present opportunities for students to deal with individual problems. As teachers use bibliotherapy in the classroom, they will help their students gain life skills and overcome personal difficulties.

ADDITIONAL MATERIALS

The classroom activity below, "Sample Lesson Plan using Bibliotherapy," demonstrates the use of bibliotherapy in a classroom. In addition, the following materials are included at the end of this chapter to assist teachers and staff:

- "Evaluating Literature for Bibliotherapy" (Handout 4.1) details criteria for evaluating the quality of books.
- A "Bibiliotherapy Summary" (Worksheet 4.1) designed to assist teachers in keeping track of good books and ideas for classroom activities.
- "Purposes and Stages of Bibliotherapy" (Overhead 4.1) summarizes basic concepts of bibliotherapy. This teaching aid could be used as an overhead or a handout in a staff/inservice training.

**CLASSROOM ACTIVITY: SAMPLE LESSON PLAN USING BIBLIOTHERAPY
(SUGGESTED AGE: GRADES 1–4)**

Topic: Dealing with reactions to trauma

Objectives

During the read-aloud story, student will be able to:

- Listen to and understand the story.
- Identify emotions of characters in the story.
- Identify emotions within self.
- Recognize appropriate ways to express emotions.

Following the read-aloud story, student will be able to:

- Use color to express emotions.
- Draw a picture using appropriate colors to express emotion.

Materials needed

For the teacher:

A *Terrible Thing Happened*, by Margaret M. Holmes (ISBN 1-55798-701-7)
Chalk or dry-erase markers and blackboard
Overhead projector, overhead, and overhead markers (if desired)

For each student:

"Expressing Our Feelings" (Worksheet 4.2)
Crayons
Blank sheet of paper

Prereading. Hold the book up so students can see the picture on the cover. Ask, "What kind of animal is this?" Acknowledge correct response. "This raccoon's name is Sherman Smith. We're going to meet Sherman in the story and learn a little about him. By raise of hand, what can you tell me about Sherman from looking at this picture?" Discuss student answers. Say, "OK. Let's read about Sherman. While we're reading, I want you to look at the pictures and think about what Sherman is feeling."

During reading. Read story. Throughout the story, pause and ask questions to increase student participation and ensure comprehension. Following are possible questions:

- p. 7—What does the expression on his face say?
- p. 9—What do you think was bothering Sherman?
- p. 12—Did your stomach ever hurt?
- p. 17—Sherman is angry. How can you tell Sherman is angry in the picture?
- p. 22–23—How did Sherman show Ms. Maple how he felt?
- p. 24—What does it look like Sherman is feeling?

- p. 25—Why do you think Sherman worried it was his fault?
- p. 27—How does Sherman feel now? Why does he feel better?
- p. 29—How do we know that Sherman is feeling better?

Postreading. After reading the story, briefly discuss what happened. Ask students the following questions:

- Tell me about Sherman.
- What were some of the feelings Sherman had?
- Who did Sherman talk to?
- What did Ms. Maple ask Sherman to do?
- How did Sherman feel after he drew the pictures and talked to someone?

After briefly discussing the plot, explain: "Sometimes bad things happen that we don't understand. And sometimes there are a lot of feelings inside of us. When Sherman didn't let his feelings out, what happened?" Acknowledge each response. Help students understand that it is okay to feel sad, mad, etc., and that sometimes, if we keep our feelings bottled up, they come out in other ways. It is important to let our feelings out in good ways.

Think–Pair–Share. Ask the following questions without giving the answers. Let the students think about each question. Write the questions on the blackboard or an overhead.

- What kinds of things do you do to show you are happy?
- What kinds of things do you do to show you are sad?
- How do people know when you are angry?

Pair each student with a partner. When you give the signal, partners share their responses. After they have had about 1 minute to share their responses with a partner, ask a few students to share with the class. Write their responses on the blackboard or overhead and reiterate: "There are many ways to show how we are feeling." Point out responses on the blackboard that refer to facial expressions. "A lot of times, you can tell how someone feels by the expression on his or her face." Hand out Worksheet 4.2, "Expressing Our Feelings" and explain: "This worksheet has pictures of people who are feeling different emotions. What feelings do you see on this page?" As students respond, give feedback.

Ask students to take out their crayons. Explain that sometimes people use color to show what they are feeling. Hold up the color red and ask, "What feeling do you think of when you see the color red?" Possible answers may be love, anger, and so on. Hold up the color blue and ask, "What feeling do you think of when you see the color blue?" Possible answers may be sad, calm, and so on. Say, "Okay, I want you to color each picture. The color you choose should go with the feeling in the picture. You choose the colors you want to use. You may use two or three colors in one picture, if you want to. In the box below each picture, identify the person's emotion."

As students are coloring their pictures, walk around the room and talk to them about what colors they are using for each emotion. After students have had enough time to color the pages, ask for examples of colors for each picture. Hold up the book again. Ask, "What did Sherman do to express his feelings about what happened?" Ask the students to think about what colors he might have used when drawing and coloring his pictures.

Tell the students to draw a picture of what happened in the story, using color to represent how they felt. After they have drawn the pictures, allow some time for discussion of their pictures. Use the *think–pair–share* format or involve the entire class in the discussion. Following the discussion, allow time for questions.

Close with the following statement: "Sometimes things happen that are hard. It's OK to feel sad and mad and upset. When we talk about it and let our feelings out in good ways, we feel better and stronger. If you need help to talk about it, it's OK to ask someone for help. Here at school there are always people who care about you and will take the time to listen."

SUGGESTED READING

Doll, B., & Doll, C. (1997). *Bibliotherapy with young people: Librarians and mental health professionals working together.* Englewood, CO: Libraries Unlimited.

Forgan, J., (2002). Using bibliotherapy to teach problem-solving. *Intervention in School and Clinic, 38*(2), 75–82.

Gladding, S. T., & Gladding, C. (1991). The ABCs of bibliotherapy for school counselors. *School Counselor, 39*(1), 7–12.

McCarty, H., & Chalmers, L. (1997). Bibliotherapy intervention and prevention. *Teaching Exceptional Children, 29,* 12–17.

Sullivan, A. K., & Strang, H. R. (2002–2003). Bibliotherapy in the classroom: Using literature to promote the development of emotional intelligence. *Childhood Education, 79*(2), 74–80.

Bibliotherapy Summary

			Excellent	Fair	Poor
Book Title		Developmental Level			
Issue Addressed		Language and Writing Style			
Author(s)		Quality of Illustrations			
Year of Publication		Life Experiences			
Publisher		Portrayal of Problems			
Address of Publisher		Problem-Solving Process			
ISBN #		Coping Skills			
Price		Characterization			
Age/Grade Level		Dialogue and Communication Skills			
# of Pages		Purpose of Emotionally Charged Scenes			
Summary of Story:		Sensitivity to Human Diversity			
		Hope and Support			

Suggested Class Activity

_____
_____
_____
_____
_____
_____
_____
_____
_____
_____
_____
_____
_____

Expressing Our Feelings

Instructions: Sometimes colors remind us of certain feelings. Color each picture to match the person's emotion. In the box below each picture, identify the person's emotion.

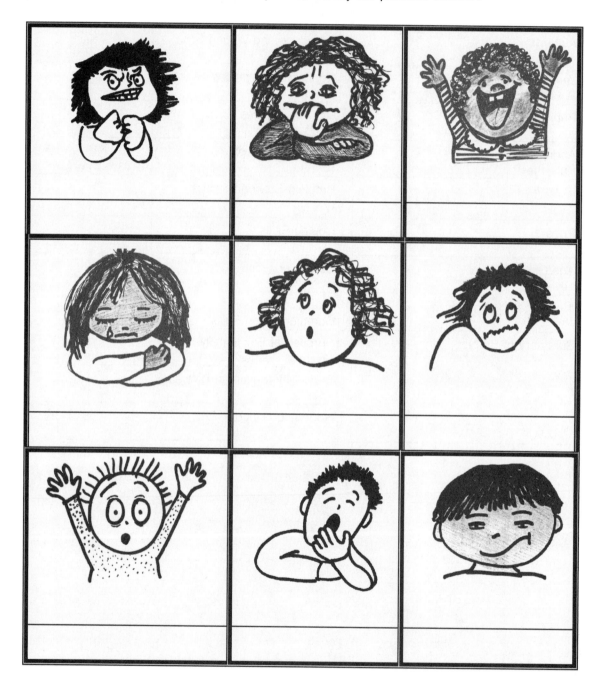

Evaluating Literature for Bibliotherapy

	Excellent	Fair	Poor/Nonexistent
Developmental Level	Language, pictures, and story are appropriate for reader's developmental level.	Inconsistent, not exactly on target with reader's developmental level.	Not appropriate for student's developmental level.
Language and Writing Style	Story is written in an easy-to-understand style. Story flows nicely and holds the reader's attention.	Writing style is uneven. Story lacks interesting details to hold the reader's attention.	Wording is clumsy, "canned," or confusing to the reader.
Quality of Illustrations	Pictures are colorful and expressive, align with the story, and hold the reader's attention.	Quality of pictures is marginal. Pictures do not accurately portray the story.	Quality of pictures is poor. Pictures do not align with the story and fail to hold the reader's interest.
Life Experiences	Portrays life in a realistic way.	Some aspects of story are realistic, others are not.	Unrealistic, not true to life.
Portrayal of Problems	Portrays problems in an honest and straightforward manner.	Problems are portrayed, but issues are sidestepped.	Unrealistic portrayal of problems and avoidance of issues.
Problem-Solving Process	Problem-solving process is explored. Characters gain insights (no "Band-Aid" solutions).	Explores process of working out problem, but solution is simplistic and arrived at too quickly.	No exploration of problem solving, reliance on "Band-Aid" solutions, or characters remain victims.
Coping Skills	Characters model healthy coping skills and problem-solving strategies.	Characters' coping skills are marginally effective or unrealistic.	Characters do not model healthy coping skills. In fact, antisocial behaviors may be promoted.
Characterization	Characters are multidimensional and show true-to-life emotions.	Characters are one-dimensional with limited emotional expression.	Characters are stereotyped and show shallow or unrealistic emotions.
Dialogue and Communication Skills	Communication skills are clearly demonstrated and dialogue holds the reader's attention.	Communication is basic and does not consistently hold the reader's interest.	Dialogue is "canned" and superficial.
Purpose of Emotionally Charged Scenes	Emotionally charged scenes serve a purpose and are not used to manipulate the reader.	Purpose of emotionally charged scenes is questionable.	Purpose of emotionally charged scenes is to entertain or to manipulate reader's emotions.
Sensitivity to Human Diversity	Sensitivity to human diversity is evident throughout the book. Pictures, story, and dialogue increase reader's understanding of others.	Story demonstrates limited sensitivity to human diversity. Story caters primarily to one cultural viewpoint.	No evidence of sensitivity to human diversity. Stereotypes fuel prejudice and cultural biases.
Hope and Support	The story gives the reader a feeling of hope and support.	The story provides limited hope and support.	The story leaves the reader with a feeling of hopelessness.

PURPOSES AND STAGES OF BIBLIOTHERAPY

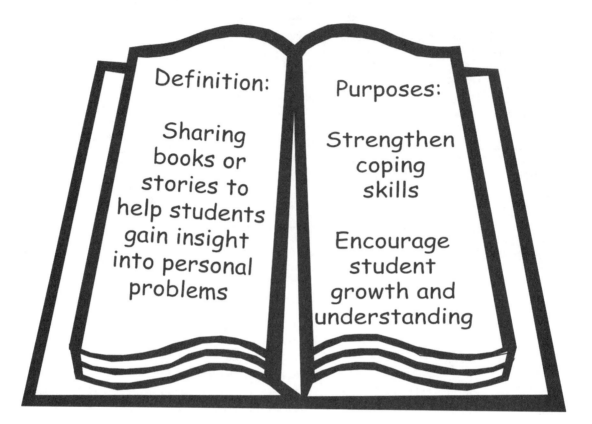

Definition:

Sharing books or stories to help students gain insight into personal problems

Purposes:

Strengthen coping skills

Encourage student growth and understanding

STAGES

Involvement: Story catches student attention.

Identification: Students identify with characters.

Catharsis: Students share characters' feelings and release emotional tension.

Insight: Students use story's lesson to help resolve personal problems.

Universalization: Students realize others have similar struggles and that they are not alone.

5

Assisting Students
with Specific Problems

Dawn Sheen, Melissa Allen Heath, Jolene Campbell,
Chrisandra Melville, *and* Bart Lyman

RESILIENCE

Resilience is defined as the ability to do well in spite of unfavorable life circumstances. Over the years researchers have defined several factors in the family, school, and community that help children thrive in adverse situations (Masten, 2001). Among these factors are safe communities, positive relationships, and success at school. Although school personnel have little control over what happens within a student's family, many things can be done to augment external assets within the school community. Fostering positive relationships between adults and students is essential. A sense of safety within the school allows students to focus more on academic work and school success increases.

Internal assets of resilient children have also been identified: positive mental health, problem-solving abilities, and social–emotional skills (Berk, 2003). Within the school setting, many opportunities arise in which school personnel can help students develop skills and characteristics that contribute to the development of successful and productive lives. Research has shown that as schools foster resilience skills—specifically social–emotional competency—students demonstrate improved academic success (Maleki & Elliot, 2002). For a more comprehensive discussion of resilience, see "Technical Assistance Sampler:

Jolene Campbell, BS, Graduate Student in School Psychology, Brigham Young University, Provo, Utah.
Chrisandra Melville, BS, Graduate Student in School Psychology, Brigham Young University, Provo, Utah.

Protective Factors/Resilience," available from *smhp.psych.ucla.edu/pdfdocs/Sampler/ Resiliency/resilien.pdf*; and *Resilient Classrooms: Creating Healthy Environments for Learning* (Doll, Zucker, & Brehm, 2004).

A review of the research related to topics discussed in this chapter provided several examples of resilience skills used to deal with adverse life situations. These skills include:

- Solving problems appropriately
- Asking for help
- Reducing stress with fun or calming activities
- Focusing on the positive
- Developing and strengthening friendships
- Learning tolerance for diversity
- Expressing feelings in appropriate ways

The remainder of the chapter contains a brief overview of important topics commonly facing students. These issues include depression, anxiety, chronic illness, difficulties making and keeping friends, divorce, problems at home, abuse, suicide, and death and grieving. Handouts and overheads for training school personnel are also included. Additionally, books and classroom activities geared toward helping students develop appropriate coping skills are described.

DEPRESSION

Depression is a state of sadness that lasts for long periods of time. When a child is grieving about something, sadness is common. If the sadness lasts for a long time or interferes a great deal with everyday functioning, it may be depression.

Many things may cause depression. The condition may be related to a chemical imbalance in the brain, stress at home or school, the death of loved ones, self-esteem issues, or the student's perception about how much he or she controls what happens in his or her life. Regardless of the cause, depressed students tend to struggle more academically.

When school personnel learn to recognize signs of depression, they can refer students to the school mental health professional. Teachers can also help students gain life skills to cope with everyday stressors. As students develop positive coping skills, risk for depression decreases (Asarnow, Jaycox, & Tompson, 2001). Adaptive coping strategies include seeking social support, solving problems, asking for help, using stress reduction techniques and focusing on the positive. Frydenberg and Lewis (1999) found that students who used positive coping strategies were more likely to have an increased sense of self-efficacy and greater academic success. They also noted that in addition to learning positive strategies, students need to be taught how to reduce maladaptive coping strategies (Frydenberg & Lewis, 2002). Maladaptive coping includes worrying, ignoring the problem, blaming oneself, avoiding other people, and engaging in destructive behaviors used to escape (e.g., drug use).

ANXIETY

Human beings have an automatic response mechanism to prepare the body for dealing with dangerous situations called the *fight-or-flight response*. When danger is perceived, the sympathetic nervous system generates a physical response. The heart beats faster; blood flow is directed toward the muscles and away from other areas of the body; breathing becomes faster; thinking becomes focused on the perceived danger; and the emotions of fear or anger surface.

Once the danger has passed, the parasympathetic nervous system takes over and the body and mind return to a normal state—but the memory of the dangerous event lingers. At times this encoding process can be highly adaptable, because the fight-or-flight response helps us recognize and be prepared for dangerous situations.

Fear is not necessarily a bad thing. Students who are afraid to play in the road because they might get hit by a car are displaying healthy fear. However, a student suffering from anxiety experiences the same physiological response as those responding to danger, but there is generally no obvious danger present. Dacey and Fiore (2002) report four central problems that anxious children face:

1. They find it harder than other children to calm themselves when they are in a stressful situation.
2. Although many of them are above average in creativity, they seldom use this ability when making plans for coping with their anxiety.
3. Even when they do have a good plan, they tend to become discouraged with it after a while and often quit trying.
4. Even when they are making progress in reducing their anxious feelings, they fail to recognize their success.

School personnel are in a key position to help students who struggle with anxiety. In addition to working with the school mental health professional to design classroom interventions, teachers can help students feel empowered. Research indicates that when students have tools, such as understanding how thoughts and feelings interact, they are better able to manage their feelings of anxiety (Velting, Setzer, & Albano, 2004). Learning to effectively solve problems is also important in conquering anxiety. School personnel, particularly teachers, can help students gain these tools and encourage them to continue trying even when it is difficult. See Overhead 5.9 to use for staff training.

CHRONIC ILLNESS

Students with chronic and serious illness struggle with a variety of issues in a school setting. Chronic absences, limited participation in school activities, teacher response to students' struggles, and peer relationships all influence the overall well-being of students with chronic illness. Teachers must be aware of the illness and side effects of medication.

Teachers and staff should review Handout 5.2 and make a plan for dealing with issues associated with chronic and serious illness. There is much a teacher can watch for and do to accommodate these students and help them feel successful as they grapple with managing their illness while at school.

DIFFICULTIES MAKING AND KEEPING FRIENDS

Positive interpersonal relationships are a necessary factor in healthy development. Relationships with parents, teachers, and friends all play a vital role in children's social development. Friends, in particular, are important to children. Unfortunately, many children struggle with making and keeping friends.

Positive friendships provide emotional support, help with problems, differing points of view, positive social experiences, opportunities to learn and practice social skills, and opportunities to practice empathy. Children without friends feel lonely, are more likely to be bullied, have lower self-esteem, have difficulties adjusting to school, and may have behavior problems.

Research indicates that students who struggle with peer relationships may be bossy, impulsive, or unkind (Coie & Dodge, 1998). They may appear judgmental of peers and insult others. Students who do not interact well with peers may also be withdrawn and not recognize or respond to attempts at friendship. Overall, difficulty making and keeping friends seems to be rooted in poor social skills. School personnel can help students who struggle with making and keeping friends by teaching them positive social skills and providing opportunities to practice these skills.

During a staff inservice, Handout 5.3, "Difficulties Making and Keeping Friends," could be reviewed. After reviewing the handout, focus on what teachers and staff can do to assist students improve social skills.

DIVORCE

Approximately half of all marriages end in divorce (Amato, 2001). Because divorce is so common, it is important to support students affected by it. In order to assist students, school personnel can increase their understanding of how students are affected by divorce.

Divorce is complicated and difficult for children and adolescents to understand; indeed, they are often confused about why parents divorce. Children wonder where they fit into the restructured family. Frequently they blame themselves for the divorce. Although children have many concerns and questions, they are hesitant to ask their parents about the divorce. Lacking information, they hold on to misconceptions and fears related to divorce. They feel alone.

Current divorce literature provides information on key issues related to children's adjustment in family transitions and how to provide appropriate support. The research findings are optimistic in regard to children's adaptability and resilience (Hetherington & Stanley-Hagan, 1999). For children experiencing parental divorce, positive outcomes are strongly correlated with availability of emotionally responsive adults and parents who provide a strong basis of emotional support (Amato, 2001). Whether their parents are divorced or together, most students benefit from learning and practicing the following skills:

- Expressing feelings in appropriate ways
- Solving problems
- Developing and strengthening friendships

Educators can help students develop and practice these skills.

PROBLEMS AT HOME

Sometimes students appear to be struggling at school, but the problem is rooted in difficulties at home. When a student's relationship with his or her parents is strained, it often leads to trouble at school. Additionally, if a parent is struggling emotionally, the child is affected. In a recent study conducted by the National Survey of American Families, findings indicated that emotional and behavioral problems are more common among children whose parents struggle with mental health issues (Brandon, 2003). Living in an environment in which a parent's emotional response is unpredictable creates fear and confusion. Children may feel responsible for fixing the problem. The constant struggle to understand unpredictable behavior and take on the impossible task of fixing the problem results in feelings of helplessness. These feelings of fear, confusion, and helplessness may be manifest in academic, social, or behavioral struggles at school.

Financial difficulties may also weigh on a student's mind. Children living in poverty are at increased risk for social–emotional and academic problems (Evans, 2004). When faced with worries and fears associated with lack of financial support, children may act out behaviorally. Their grades may deteriorate, and they may be rejected by peers. With poverty often comes neglect or abuse. Students struggling to find hope in such circumstances benefit greatly from supportive, caring adults who provide a sense of stability in an otherwise chaotic world.

Through a series of interviews with impoverished children, Percy (2003) found that feeling loved and having supportive friendships were essential to each child's sense of well-being. Although school professionals do not directly offer the same friendship as a student's peer, they can give support and love. Teachers can also teach social skills to students who do not have any positive friendships. Opportunities to practice these new social skills can be provided in the rich social environment of the school.

ABUSE

There are three major categories of abuse: sexual, physical, and emotional. Teachers and staff are required to report all *suspected* abuse to the proper authorities, typically Child Protective Services or the Department of Human Services. If you suspect abuse, report it.

Clearly report facts as facts and suspicion as suspicion. There are national telephone hotlines open 24 hours a day. Toll-free numbers are listed in phone books. Most schools have an outlined routine for reporting suspected abuse. Some schools may require a written report to be filed with the school nurse or principal. It is important to know your school's policy and to follow its guidelines.

In response to abuse, children may feel guilt, shame, isolation, and fear. Feeling powerless, they may also feel hopeless and depressed. Some children may consider suicide or running away to escape the abuse; some may suffer with high levels of anxiety that render them easily startled and sensitive to loud noises or touch.

Teachers and staff must consult with mental health professionals to determine how to adapt their classroom to the needs of a student with a history of abuse. The goal is to reduce stress and anxiety, creating an environment in which the student feels safe and secure. Suggested interventions may be as simple as seating the student in the back corner of the classroom, where he or she can see everything and feel more in control. Other students may feel more secure being seated next to the teacher's desk or near the door or window. Specific situations may require different strategies, depending on the student's worries and fears. In extreme cases of anxiety, the student may need a hall pass to visit with the school counselor.

SUICIDE

Suicide is the eighth leading cause of death in the United States. For youth and adults ages 15–34, it is the third leading cause of death. On average, 84 Americans commit suicide every day. Over the last four decades, suicide rates among youth have increased drastically (U.S. Department of Health and Human Services, 2001). It is essential that school personnel know the risk factors and warning signs of suicide.

Some risk factors include adjustment problems; lack of social connections; feelings of extreme shame, anxiety, or depression; alcohol or drug use; a sudden change in personality; or participation in dangerous activities. Other considerations include a history of suicidal behavior, a loss of interest in life, or a preoccupation with death. Overtly preparing for death by giving away favorite possessions or discussing suicidal plans is a sign that a suicide attempt may be imminent.

When teachers and staff notice warning signs of suicide, they must take time to speak with the at-risk student. A suicidal student is more likely to confide in a teacher he or she sees everyday than to seek help from a counselor he or she has never met. If a student discloses a desire to commit suicide to you, remain calm and listen. Express concern for the student's safety and suggest meeting with the school mental health professional. You might say, "I care about you and want to get someone to help us. When you care about someone, you don't want them to hurt themselves. I want to help you."

In addition to observing student behavior and responding to clear warning signs, teachers can incorporate activities into classroom curriculum that are geared toward suicide prevention. The best defense is a good offense. Research shows that students who are depressed are at higher risk for committing suicide (Brock & Sandoval, 1997; Sandoval & Brock, 1996). Helping students acquire coping skills can help stop the problem before it starts. Social isolation also plays a role in suicidal thinking. Assisting students to find social connections by improving interpersonal skills is also helpful.

DEATH AND GRIEVING

When a student experiences loss, he or she generally goes through a cycle of mourning that involves several stages (Kübler-Ross, 1969). It is important for school personnel to be aware of how a grieving student may react as well as what he or she needs in order to cope with the loss. Following are the stages of the mourning cycle:

- *Sadness*: Sadness is a common reaction to loss. Children may withdraw or show less interest in activities they previously enjoyed. Over time, the initial sadness should decrease as the child moves into other stages of grieving.
- *Denial*: In response to loss, children may experience denial for several reasons. First, it is difficult to accept that a loved one is not coming back. Additionally, many unpleasant emotions accompany death. Difficulty tolerating intense emotion causes children to move into a fantasy world where they do not have to deal with death. This reaction is OK; however, if the child does not come back to reality, problems may result. Talking to the child about the person who died and recalling positive, loving, and happy experiences with him or her is helpful.
- *Guilt*: Children may think that the death is their fault, or that they could have prevented it. Adults can remove this misperceived responsibility by repeatedly reassuring the child that the death was not their fault and that there is nothing they could have done to stop it.
- *Anger*: The root of anger is often chaotic emotion that needs to be understood and expressed. Any change in life brings uncomfortable feelings. Emotions related to loss can be particularly confusing. Acting out that confusion via disruptive behavior is common. Adults can help by understanding where the anger comes from and having patience. Coaching the child in recognizing and expressing each emotion is also helpful.
- *Shame/stigma*: Children want to believe that they are like everyone else, that they blend into the crowd. When a loved one dies, it sets them apart as different. They may also feel embarrassed by the attention of adults paying condolences. When they experience a loss, they may feel different. Being different feels shameful. Involving a child with a group of peers who has experienced similar losses may be helpful.
- *Acceptance*: As children who have experienced loss reach different stages in their development, they will recycle through the first steps of mourning. Children go through many milestones during which the missing presence of a loved one is noticed. Typically, children come gradually to accept the death but continue to remember their loss, even into adulthood (Fitzgerald, 1992).

As the mourning student cycles through each stage, there is much school personnel can do to help. When speaking with a student who is grieving, it is important to acknowledge the loss. Being sensitive to the situation and authentic when expressing feelings are essential to building and maintaining a relationship of trust. Avoid asking questions to satisfy curiosity, but reassure the student that you are there if he or she wants to talk. Students who have experienced loss may need to reminisce about their loved one. Allow them to do so when ready.

STAFF TRAINING HANDOUTS

School mental health professionals are in a key position to disseminate information regarding student reactions to both minor developmental transitions and major events. As teachers and staff meet during faculty meetings and inservice trainings, mental health professionals can provide quick facts about specific crises as well as more in-depth crisis training geared toward each staff or faculty member's role in the school. Garet, Porter, Desimone, Birman, and Yoon suggest the following strategies when developing effective professional development programs (cited in Elliot, Kratochwill, & Roach, 2003):

- Concentrate on adding to participants' knowledge base.
- Encourage active learning.
- Be consistent and coherent during training over time.
- Set goals to bring about meaningful change.
- Foster collaboration by involving all teachers and staff in the school.
- Allow adequate training time to accomplish established goals.

Handouts and overheads that can be used during staff training are provided at the end of the chapter. Some of these handouts pertain to staff education, and some to student education. Presenting information related to crisis intervention is essential. From a brief summary of handouts and overheads to more elaborate cooperative learning activities, topics can be covered in a variety of ways. Be creative as you foster learning among faculty and staff.

Handout and Overhead Topics

- Depression (Handout 5.1)
- Anxiety (Overhead 5.9)
- Chronic and serious illness (Handout 5.2)
- Difficulties making and keeping friends (Handout 5.3)
- Divorce (Handout 5.4)
- Abuse (Handouts 5.5 and 5.6; Overheads 5.1–5.3)
- Suicide (Handout 5.7; Overheads 5.4 and 5.5)
- Death and Grief (Handout 5.8–5.10; Overhead 5.6)

BIBLIOTHERAPY ACTIVITIES

The following suggestions for books and activities can be copied and distributed to teachers and staff for use in the classroom. As part of training faculty and staff, school mental health professionals could also read suggested books and model the activities.

Suggested Books

- *When Addie Was Scared* (Bibliotherapy Summary 5.1)
- *Joey Pigza Swallowed the Key* (Bibliotherapy Summary 5.2)
- *How to Lose All Your Friends* (Bibliotherapy Summary 5.3)
- *When Zachary Beaver Came to Town* (Bibliotherapy Summary 5.4)
- *My Louisiana Sky* (Bibliotherapy Summary 5.5)
- *Define "Normal"* (Bibliotherapy Summary 5.6)
- *Gettin' through Thursday* (Bibliotherapy Summary 5.7)
- *Money Hungry* (Bibliotherapy Summary 5.8)
- *Ramona and Her Father* (Bibliotherapy Summary 5.9)
- *Lilly's Purple Plastic Purse* (Bibliotherapy Summary 5.10)
- *Is It Right to Fight?* (Bibliotherapy Summary 5.11)

CLASSROOM ACTIVITIES

Activities emphasizing resilience skills are described in the following material. They are designed to be used in both small-group situations by a mental health professional as well as by a teacher in classroom settings. Although teachers should not therapeutically counsel students, they can teach many skills related to resilience. Figure 5.1 indicates which activities may be helpful for specific topics conditions/problems covered in this chapter.

HAPPY HARRY, SAD SALLY

Objective: Students will connect how thoughts influence feelings.
Materials needed

Picture of an optical illusion
Pictures of situations that could evoke different emotions
White erase markers

Think–pair–share
Think: Hold up picture of an optical illusion. Tell students to think about what they see for 30 seconds, then ask them to pay attention to how they feel about what they are looking at.

ACTIVITY	TOPICS	Page #	Depression	Anxiety	Chronic illness	Friendship problems	Divorce	Abuse	Suicide	Problems at home	General coping skills
Happy Harry, Sad Sally	Thought, feeling, action connection	85	×	×	×	×	×	×	×	×	×
We Aren't "Bugged"!	General coping skills	87	×	×	×	×	×	×	×	×	×
Monster Power	Overcoming fear	87		×	×	×	×	×	×	×	×
Tower of Tolerance	Tolerance, cooperation	88			×	×	×			×	×
Divorce Feelings: Change	Coping with change	89					×				
Divorce Feelings: Parent Talk	Dealing with feelings	90					×				
Defining Group Rules	Rules for groups	90					×				
Backpack Activity	Dealing with feelings	91	×	×	×	×	×	×	×	×	×
Make Me Laugh Game	Dealing with feelings	93	×	×		×					×
Homemade Gak	General coping	93	×	×	×	×	×	×	×	×	×
Masks	Dealing with feelings	94	×	×	×	×	×	×	×	×	×
Ice Cream Get to Know You Game	Getting to know you	97	×	×	×	×	×	×	×	×	×
I Like People Who . . .	Getting to know you	97	×	×	×	×	×	×	×	×	×
Name Game	Getting to know you	97	×	×	×	×	×	×	×	×	×
Lifting Activity	Teamwork	98	×	×	×	×	×	×	×	×	×
ABC Scavenger Hunt	Teamwork	98	×	×	×	×	×	×	×	×	×
Linked Elbow Stand	Working together	99	×	×	×	×	×	×	×	×	×
Communication Tennis	Communication skills	99	×	×	×	×	×	×	×	×	×
Eye Contact Ball Game	Communication skills	99	×	×	×	×	×	×	×	×	×
"I Feel" Messages	Communication skills, emotions	100	×	×	×	×	×	×	×	×	×
Tangled Arms Game	Problem solving	100	×	×	×	×	×	×	×	×	×
Problem Solving	Problem solving	100	×	×	×	×	×	×	×	×	×
Around the Table Compliments	Self-image, giving and receiving compliments	101	×	×	×	×	×	×	×	×	×
Snowball fight	Self-image, giving and receiving compliments	102	×	×	×	×	×	×	×	×	×
Quality chain	Self-image	102	×	×	×	×	×	×	×	×	×

FIGURE 5.1. Suggested activities, topics addressed, and conditions/problems to which they apply.

Pair: After about 15–30 seconds, have students pair up with a partner and ask: "What did you see? What did you think of when you saw it? How did you feel when you looked at it?"

Share: Ask the class: "What did you see? Was it the same or different from what your partner saw? If your partner saw something different, were you able to see it? How did your thoughts and feelings change about what you were looking at when you saw it differently?" Explain: "Often what we perceive determines what we think and how we feel. What we think and how we feel then determine how we may act." On the blackboard, draw a large triangle and label the three sides: *thoughts*, *feelings*, and *actions*.

Happy/sad thoughts

Draw two faces on the blackboard, one happy face (Happy Harry) and one sad face (Sad Sally). Explain that the names of these two people are Happy Harry and Sad Sally. Tell students that in *every* situation, Harry is happy, but Sally is sad. Divide students into groups of four and randomly assign each group to one of the two categories: Happy Harry or Sad Sally.

Say: "I am going to show you several pictures. With each picture, I want you to discuss why the situation in the picture would make you feel happy or sad. If you are 'Happy Harry,' talk about what thoughts would make you feel happy about the situation. If you are 'Sad Sally,' what thoughts would make you feel sad about the picture?" After presenting each picture and permitting time for group discussion, ask a spokesperson from each group to share his or her group's thoughts. Make a list of happy thoughts under the picture of Happy Harry, and sad thoughts under the picture of Sad Sally.

Point out that what we think can determine what we feel, and that what we feel often determines how we act. Acknowledge that we all experience situations that are sad or difficult, and that it is important to recognize those feelings. Explain that it is possible to have a positive perspective even when things are difficult. Sometimes we may feel sad or angry for a really long time and not know why. We may not know what is causing the sadness. When this happens, it is important to talk to someone and get help. That's OK. When we are able to identify happy or sad thoughts tied to our feelings and actions, we better understand ourselves and others. Close the lesson with Worksheet 5.1, "Thoughts Connect with Feelings."

WE AREN'T "BUGGED"!

This activity (Worksheets 5.2 and 5.3) can be used with either a classroom of students or with a small group of students. Boys will especially like this activity because it uses characteristics of insects to teach students about perseverance and dealing with less-than-ideal situations. Discuss the interesting facts about the insects and then draw comparisons with real-life situations. What can we learn from the insects?

MONSTER POWER

Have students talk about what scares them and why. Talk about how fears can often be represented with images. *What images represent fear?* Explain that today we will use the image of a monster to represent fear. Using magazines in whatever way they would like, ask students to create a monster that represents the fear (i.e., choosing images from the magazine that represent parts of their fear). Show an example. When students finish creating the monster, talk about what makes the monster so big. Ask students what they can do about those parts. Brainstorm a list of empowering activities. On the other side of the page, have students create a second collage depicting themselves as bigger than the monster. Include pictures of what they can do to fight the monster. Have students choose one thing on the previously created list that they will do this week to feel empowered.

TOWER OF TOLERANCE

Materials needed

Straws
Masking tape
Paper lunch bags
Blindfolds

For each group provide 20 straws, several feet of masking tape, three paper lunch bags, and one blindfold.

The task

Groups of students use straws and masking tape to build what they hope will be the tallest tower in the class. The towers must be sturdy enough to withstand being moved to the front of the room and placed on a desk. The teacher will then create an earthquake or great wind storm to make the towers fall. The tallest tower left standing wins.

The process

Divide students into groups of four and assign a number (1–4) to each person in the group. Give each group the required supplies. Instruct students not to touch the supplies until you tell them to do so. Explain the task to students and check for understanding.

Before beginning tower construction, give students 5 minutes to plan how they will construct their tower. Make sure they know to begin actual construction only *after* you give the signal. After 5 minutes, instruct all Number 1 students to place both hands inside a lunch bag and have a fellow group member wrap tape around their wrists to secure the bags. They are not to use their hands. All Number 2 students should do the same, but only placing their dominant hand in a lunch bag. Number 3 students are told they cannot speak, and Number 4 students are blindfolded. Instruct groups that for this activity, every member of the group must participate. Students who do not follow the rules will be disqualified. It is up to group members to decide how to include everyone. They will have 10–15 minutes to complete the tower.

Wait for groaning and complaining to cease, then give the signal to begin. Monitor students to ensure that they are working with their assigned limitations appropriately. When there are 2 minutes left, tell students to start wrapping it up. When the time is up, have students stop working. One student from each group should bring their tower to the front of the room. The towers are tested simultaneously for earthquake and wind safety. The tallest tower left standing wins.

Discussion

After completing the activity, follow up by discussing students' experiences. Help students recognize the importance of working together, including others, and looking past outward limitations. Suggested questions include:

- What was your limitation?
- How did you feel about your limitation?
- Did you feel included in your group?
- What did other group members do to help you feel included?
- What did you do to help other group members feel included?
- What was difficult about this activity?
- Why?
- Did you feel you had something to contribute to the group?
- Why or why not?
- What would you do differently in the future?
- How can this activity apply to other situations in school?
- How can this activity apply to other situations in life?

Activities for Mental Health Professionals

TOPIC: DIVORCE FEELINGS: CHANGE

Materials needed

Picture of a puppy

Procedure

Show students the picture of a puppy. Ask: "How does a newborn puppy change over time?" Discuss.

Explain: "Families can also change. Divorce changes a family. Divorce means 'no longer married.' Even though this is a big change, some things are still the same. Parents love their children. This does not change. Parents will always love you, even when their feelings for each other change."

Draw pictures of things that change in families after parents separate or divorce. Some changes may include moving to another home, not seeing Father (or Mother) as often, more (or less) crying, more (or less) arguing, not as much money, more quiet time, more watching TV, more (or less) eating out at McDonald's and so on.

Summary: "Changes are different for each family. But one thing remains the same. [Flip poster over and draw a big heart.] Parents love their kids. [Write the word *family* in the center of the heart.] And kids have love in their hearts for their family."

TOPIC: DIVORCE FEELINGS: PARENT TALK

After playing "Make Me Laugh Game" (p. 93), have the following discussion (best used in a divorce group). Discuss: "How do you think parents feel about divorce? Parents may be angry with each other after they separate. They may say mean things to their kids about each other. Kids need to stay out of their parents' problems. When parents argue, it is about adult stuff. Kids don't like to hear bad stuff about their parents. It hurts to hear bad stuff. Sometimes parents try to get kids involved by having them give messages to the other parent. It's not the kid's job to send messages from one parent to the other. Parents need to talk directly to each other."

Activity: Drawing "feelings about divorce"

Give each student Worksheet 5.5 and crayons. Ask how kids might feel about divorce. Read the directions at the top of the worksheet. Allow about 5 minutes for the students to draw their pictures. Encourage students to share their ideas.

Discuss: "How do kids deal with their feelings? How can kids release anger in a healthy way? Who can they talk to when they are upset?" Close the discussion with the "Divorce Worksheet" (5.4). Review the students' responses and clarify any misconceptions.

Additional Activities

DEFINING GROUP RULES

Setting limits provides a secure and comfortable atmosphere for students. It is imperative to outline the basic rules during the first group meeting. Rules should be easy to understand; the number of rules should be limited to five or less; and rules should be stated with a positive slant. For instance, rules should inform students about what they should do, rather than warn them about what they should not do. Pictures or visual cues will help students remember rules. Rules should be posted and referred to frequently (see Overhead 5.7). Recommended rules and discussion may include:

1. *Listen when others talk.* "Each of you will have a turn to talk. A good listener does not interrupt or talk over someone else's comments. If you want to make a comment, wait for your turn when everyone is listening."

2. *Keep hands and feet to self.* "We respect other group members' personal space."

3. *Support each other.* "Use kind words. Think about how your words make others feel. Use a "thumbs up" sign to show your support."

4. *Share or "pass."* "Each group member has the right to talk when it is his or her turn, or to be quiet and say 'pass' if he or she does not want to talk. Our thoughts and feelings are traveling at different speeds. We must be comfortable with going at our own speed. It is OK for each of us to go at our own speed."

5. *Respect others.* "Respect for ourselves and others is the most important group rule. When we respect someone, we value his or her thoughts and words, and we want that person to feel comfortable and accepted. When a student talks about his or her feelings, we listen and try to understand him or her. We don't laugh or make fun of the person. What is said in the group stays in the group. We feel safe in our group when we know others will

not tease us. We show respect by not talking about group members' feelings outside of group, in the classroom, or on the playground. However, no matter what, you can always talk with your teacher or parents if something scares you or feels uncomfortable. Although our group discussion is not a secret, we want to show respect for others' feelings by not gossiping or storytelling about our group."

Activities Related to Feelings

BACKPACK ACTIVITY

This activity is designed to be adapted for many situations with children or adults. It has been used effectively to explain the benefits of healthfully releasing angry or sad feelings. Students seem to grasp the concepts better after experiencing the visual and perceptual metaphor of the backpack and canned food. The material with quotation marks can be used as a partial script for the activity.

Materials needed

> Backpack
> Canned food (variety of shapes and sizes; cover labels with plain paper)
> Marker

Procedure

Gather group into a circle or other arrangement where everyone can see the demonstration. Have cans of food stacked or lined up on a table. Explain: "This backpack represents our bodies, and the cans represent mad or sad feelings. Sometimes these feelings are small like this can. [Hold up a small can.] Sometimes feelings are big like this can. [Hold up a large can.] The small can represents something that may happen every day, like being cut off in the lunch line. The big can represents something more serious, like when your pet dies." Ask students to share situations that bring out mad or sad feelings. Write their examples on can labels that correspond in size to the seriousness of the situation. As each can is labeled, add it to the backpack.

After all cans have been placed in the bag, pass it around the group for each student to lift. Ask: "Would it be possible to participate in activities you enjoy carrying such a heavy bag? Of your favorite activities, which would be the most difficult to do?" Possible answers might include swimming, playing the piano, baseball, dancing, playing video games. Explain: "When we carry mad and sad feelings inside, it is a heavy burden. Just like heavy cans, these feelings may keep us from enjoying things we usually like. They can keep us from doing our best in school. They may make us not want to play. Hard feelings might also make us feel cranky, so that we respond to others differently than we normally would. Maybe we are impatient with a friend or parent. This is our body's way of telling us that we have feelings deep inside that need to be let out."

Explain: "There are helpful and unhelpful ways to deal with tough feelings." Give examples of each. "Many people find that when they are mad, they have extra energy. Exercising can be a helpful way to use that extra energy. At other times, having quiet alone time or talking to a good friend is most helpful. When getting feelings out, it is important to follow two rules: (1) Don't hurt people (self or others), and (2) don't hurt things. Using energy to destroy things or hurt others is not a healthy way to express feelings."

Ask students for examples of expressing feelings in ways that follow these two rules. For each healthy idea, take one can out of the backpack.

Reassure students: "All of us have different feelings from time to time. However, you can decide how you will react to your feelings. You can make sure you aren't holding them inside and carrying them around longer than you need to. When we have difficult feelings, it is better to deal with them in a healthy way than to keep them inside."

Additional discussion for specific situations

Sensitivity to others' needs: Explain: The backpack activity can also help us understand others and be more sensitive to their needs. Maybe someone's bag is heavy with lots of feelings stuffed inside. Unaware of that person's heavy backpack, we might say something that hurts his or her feelings. This adds another can to his or her heavy backpack. Because the person is already exhausted from carrying such a heavy load, he or she might lash out and dump the heavy load of feelings on us.

"Another example is when Mom asks John to take out the trash. Taking out the trash is not fun, but usually John does the chore without complaining. However, today John complains and stomps his foot in anger. Mom might not know that John had a bad day at school. He got in a fight with his best friend. His backpack is full to overflowing. Because he already has feelings stuffed inside, he becomes overly upset about taking the trash out, complains, and stomps his foot in anger.

"It is important to be understanding of others' feelings. When other people overreact to something we do or say, they might already have a full backpack. We need to be careful not to add more cans to someone's backpack. We also need to be careful about overreacting to others when our backpack is full. It makes sense to keep our backpack as empty as possible."

Suicide: In the case of suicide, school staff must be particularly sensitive to students' reactions. Students will have a difficult time understanding why someone would commit suicide. The backpack activity helps students understand how stress builds over time when feelings are kept stuffed inside. The backpack activity provides a basis for discussion of healthy ways to deal with stress.

Emphasize: "Sometimes people with heavy cans in their backpack forget about healthy ways to reduce stress. Their backpacks were full, but they did not see any other way to reduce the load. They were not thinking of anything else except getting rid of the heavy backpack. Their solution, suicide, was not a good solution. It was a permanent solution to a temporary problem. It is very important to remember: There are always other choices. There are healthy ways to reduce your load."

Brainstorm and discuss healthy ways to deal with sadness and anger. Ask students to pick the ideas that work best for them. Emphasize: "Find support in friends and adults who care. A heavy load is much lighter when someone helps us carry it."

MAKE ME LAUGH GAME

Ask students if another person can *make* them feel a certain way. Ask for a volunteer who thinks that others cannot make him or her laugh. The volunteer is seated in a chair at the front of the group. Another student is selected to take a turn at trying to make the volunteer laugh without touching him or her. You could also pair the students; one student would take the role of not laughing and the other would try to make his or her partner laugh.

Discuss: "Our feelings belong to us. Others can't make us feel a certain way unless we give them permission to do so." Discuss healthy ways to release our feelings. Make sure to follow the two rules: Don't hurt people and don't hurt things. Review the backpack activity if the group needs more discussion about expressing feelings.

Discuss: "How do kids deal with feelings? How can kids release anger in a healthy way? Who can they talk to when they are upset?"

HOMEMADE GAK

There is a saying: "Children are like water; if they aren't in a container, they are all over the place." This activity can represent several metaphorical meanings.

Materials needed

Two mixing bowls
Wire whisk
Food coloring (optional)
1 cup (7.625 fl. oz.) Elmer's multipurpose white glue
1 cup cold tap water
1 cup warm tap water
4 tsp. "20 Mule Team Borax"

Procedure

Have students prepare the gak ingredients in two separate mixing bowls. In the first bowl they should mix 1 cup cold water with 1 cup (7.625 fl. oz.) Elmer's multipurpose white glue. (*Note*: Do not use Elmer's *school* glue, use regular Elmer's glue.) They mix the glue and cold water by stirring and squishing the mixture with a wire whisk or, for a wonderfully messy tactile experience, they can mix it with their bare hands.

In the second bowl students should mix 1 cup of warm water with 4 teaspoons of "20 Mule Team Borax," a laundry powder used for soaking stains and removing odors. After both mixtures are sufficiently stirred, students should pour the bowl of warm water/Borax into the bowl of cold water/glue. Immediately, the mixture begins to gel. Students should thoroughly squish the slimy white ingredients for 5–10 minutes, incorporating the solid material into the liquid. At first the solid and the liquid are difficult to integrate. Students should continue squishing the material with their bare hands. Eventually the liquid and solid combine to form a gelatinous mass.

Remind students that the gak recipe makes something unlike any of its individual ingredients. Students will question what they are making, particularly as they squish the slimy ingredients with their bare hands. However, in the end, students are very pleased with their concoction. At the conclusion of the activity, emphasize these points: "You followed directions. You stuck to it. You did not give up. The final mixture is very different from the ingredients. Gak is something new and unique."

Give a handful of gak to each student. Watch for their discovery of the properties of gak. Note the material's consistency. Gak will slide through their fingers if students are not continuously squeezing it. Similarly, when a student's emotions are out of control and "running all over the place," others (teachers, parents, and friends) assist in helping him or her regain control. Discuss when a person's emotions might become "out of control." What happens when emotions are not contained? Assist students in understanding the need for counselors, school psychologists, parents, and teachers to help maintain order and control situations, particularly during a crisis. Discuss strategies for assisting others to regain control of their emotions and identify strategies for maintaining self-control.

Gak friendship activity

Gak can also be used to demonstrate how different things join together, making something that is totally different and fun. Making gak can represent building a new friendship. Explain: "No two people have the same personality. When two people come together, they bring out different qualities in each other. Friends do not need to be exactly alike. In making gak, the warm water is different from the cold water. Friends can be very different from one another, and their individual characteristics can complement each other."

Discuss personality differences and how two different qualities may compliment each other. Some examples include shy versus friendly and outgoing; artistic and creative versus practical minded; quiet versus talkative; athletic versus studious; passive versus active; serious versus humorous; calm versus emotional; and supportive versus directive.

DRAWING ACTIVITY: MASKS

This activity is adjusted for two age groups: ages 5–11 and 12–18. Use the stories and accompanying worksheets identified for the appropriate age group. Give each student a worksheet (Worksheet 5.6 for ages 5–11 and Worksheet 5.7 for ages 12–18) and a pencil.

Purpose: To increase students' understanding of emotions and emotional expression. Stories and the accompanying drawing activity demonstrate the difference between external expression of feelings and the true feelings underlying those expressions.

Ages 5–11

Story 1: "Salina is in the second grade. She looks very happy today. She is smiling. Draw a smile on the top circle. But Salina's smile does not show how she is feeling inside. Salina is angry with her teacher because her teacher made her redo a math worksheet. Salina is trying very hard to look happy. She does not want her teacher to know how angry she is about the math worksheet. She is trying to have a good attitude. Draw an angry face on the bottom circle. The teacher sees the happy face, but Salina has an angry face inside."

Question: "Why does Salina show a happy face on the outside when her face on the inside is angry?"

Explain: "When we wear a mask, we put on a face for everyone to see. The mask that people see looks different than how we are really feeling on the inside. Sometimes it feels uncomfortable to keep our feelings stuffed inside. When we hide our feelings, others might not know how we really feel. Sometimes it is hard to know how someone feels on the inside."

Story 2: Michael is in first grade. He thinks his mother and father are getting a divorce. They fight a lot. He hurts inside when he hears them fight. His mother and father get very angry with each other. Sometimes they yell and throw things at each other. He cries when he is alone in his room at night. Michael wants to pretend that all of this is not happening. When he is at school he *never* wants to talk about his family. He wants to pretend that everything is OK. Today he is very tired. His parents fought last night after he went to bed. They thought he was sleeping. He was not sleeping. He was crying and afraid in his room. He felt alone. Right now he is sitting at his school desk. He is smiling and trying hard to pretend that everything is OK. He is trying to forget the feelings inside. Inside he is tired and very sad. His teacher and friends see Michael's mask, his smiling face. But he is very sad inside. Draw a happy face on the other circle at the top of the worksheet. This is Michael's mask on the outside. Now go down to the bottom of the page and draw a sad face on the bottom circle. This is how Michael feels inside. This is how he *really* feels."

Directions: Fold the worksheet in half on the dotted line so that the masks, the top circles, hide the bottom circles. When the worksheet is folded, hold the paper so that the masks are on top. The masks hide the bottom circles that are folded underneath.

Discussion and questions:

- "Michael wished he had happy feelings inside all of the time."
- "Would you like to have happy feelings inside all of the time?"
- "Everybody wishes for happy feelings, but no one has happy feelings all of the time."
- "Do you think Michael will let someone see his true feelings?"
- "What do you think would happen if someone saw Michael's hidden feelings?"
- "Who could Michael talk with about his sad feelings?"

Conclusion: "It is important to know the difference between inside and outside feelings. When people see our mask, it is hard for them to know how we really feel inside. If we hold things inside, sometimes our feelings come out in other ways. We might get very upset over something small, like dropping our book or tripping up the stairs. Although we can wear a mask, the feelings are still there inside. It is important to know who we can talk to about our inside feelings."

Ages 12–18

Directions: Draw a happy, joking face in the first top circle, the mask.

Story: "Miguel is in eighth grade. Everyone thinks he is cool. His clothes are his own style, not some preppy stuff from a magazine. Whenever he talks, everyone pays attention. It's not like he tries to be this way; he just is. Miguel never gets upset. He is always joking. In class the teachers think he is disrespectful and rude, but he makes even them laugh sometimes. He turns every situation into a joke. That is Miguel on the outside, laughing and joking. That is the mask he wears.

"His mask is covering his true feelings inside, his feelings of worry and fear. Although he appears happy, Miguel worries on the inside. He feels scared for his older brother, Tony. Last week Tony was in a motorcycle accident. It was serious. Tony hurt his back really badly and the doctors say he might be paralyzed. No one knows for sure yet. The hospital bills and doctor bills are very high, and Miguel's parents are fighting about money. They don't have insurance. Miguel is very worried and scared about Tony and his family's money problems."

Directions: Draw a sad and worried face in the bottom circle to the far left.

Information and questions: "Miguel, like every other kid, would like to feel great all the time. He wished he *never* had problems. Problems are no fun. But everyone, even those who look happy all of the time, has problems. Problems bring sad feelings, angry feelings, confused feelings, and many other feelings. No one has happy feelings all of the time."

- "Do you think it is hard for Miguel to let others see his true feelings inside?"
- "Why is it difficult for Miguel to show his true feelings?"
- "Do you think Miguel could talk to someone about his worries and fears?"
- "What do you think would happen if Miguel talked to his friends about how he really felt?"

Discussion about feelings: "It is important to know the difference between our true inner feelings and the feelings we let others see, our mask. If we only let others see our mask, it is difficult for them to know how we feel inside. It takes a lot of energy to keep feelings stuffed inside.

"Sometimes our inner feelings come out in other ways. For instance, we might get very upset over small things, like breaking our pencil lead or tripping up the stairs. Keeping our feelings stuffed inside makes it harder for us to deal with the little things that happen.

"There are many healthy ways to express inner feelings. Artists express their inner feelings in their artwork. Athletes run really fast or play a very rough game of football to let off steam.

"Sometimes people let their inner feelings out when they are alone. They might sing their favorite song really loud or cry quietly in their bed at night. Some people write beautiful poetry or write in their journal. Other ways to express feelings include the way we dress, the way we decorate our bedroom, how we style our hair, the type of music we listen to, the books we choose to read, and the words we speak.

"Movie directors express their feelings by directing actors in emotional scenes. We can feel those feelings as we watch the movie. Although no one feels exactly the same way we do, we can share similar feelings. In the dark movie theatre, we might cry when we see something sad, like when someone is dying or when someone is alone. Feelings have a wide range of intensity and variety.

"Although we have control over which mask we choose to wear and which mask covers our feelings inside, the feelings are still there. It is important to know who we can talk to about our true feelings and how we can express our feelings in healthy ways. Our feelings give us energy. It is important to use this energy in a healthy way."

Directions for drawing activity: "The top of this worksheet has two other circles to represent the masks kids sometimes wear to hide their true inner feelings. The two other bottom circles represent the true inner feelings that the masks are hiding. Draw two masks in the top circles and then draw the feelings the masks are hiding in the two bottom circles. Think of a situation to go along with each set (the mask and corresponding bottom circle)." Allow approximately 5 minutes to complete the activity.

"Fold the worksheet in half on the dotted line so that the masks, the top circles, hide the bottom circles. When the worksheet is folded, hold the paper so that the masks are on top. The masks hide the bottom circles that are folded underneath."

Discussion: Ask for volunteers to discuss the situations represented by their drawings.

Conclusion: "Remember, it is important to know the difference between our true inner feelings and the feelings we let others see, our mask. If we only let others see our mask, it is difficult for them to know how we feel inside. It takes a lot of energy to keep feelings stuffed inside. It is important to share our true feelings with people we trust."

Getting to Know You Activities

ICE CREAM GET TO KNOW YOU GAME

Ask students to sit in a circle. Each student introduces themselves by sharing the following information: name, birthday, grade in school, and a favorite flavor of ice cream.

I LIKE PEOPLE WHO . . .

Form a circle of chairs with one less chair than the number of students in the group. One student stands in the middle of the circle and says: "I like people who. . . . " The student adds a trait or description to complete the sentence. For instance, the student might say "I like people who have brown eyes" or "I like people who have shoes with buckles." Anyone who fits the description jumps up and changes chairs with others who also fit the description. The student in the middle of the circle also tries to find an open chair. The one student left standing goes into the center of the circle, and the game continues.

NAME GAME

Have students sit in a circle. Students begin by introducing themselves by name. You begin clapping a rhythm cycle by hitting your knees twice, clapping twice, and snapping twice. After the second snap, you call a name. The person whose name was called must call another name before the rhythm cycle is done (i.e., before second snap). If the child does not call a name before everyone snaps the second time, he or she is out. The game continues until most students are out.

Teamwork Activities

LIFTING ACTIVITY (ALL AGES)

Explain: "When things seem impossible or overwhelming, we need to remember the strength we gain from unity." Ask one student to sit on a table or desk. Ask another student to lift the student on the table/desk with one finger. This seems impossible! It *is* impossible with only one finger providing the power. Now ask 15 students to come forward and, as a group, to each use one finger to lift the student on the table/desk. Ask students to lift the table/desk 1 inch off the ground. Then ask students to state in one sentence what they learned from the lifting activity. Possible lessons might include:

"A little help from many friends goes a long way."
"Many hands make heavy work lighter."
"When everyone joins in, amazing things can be accomplished."
"We are stronger when we work together as a group."

ABC SCAVENGER HUNT (AGES 8 AND OLDER)

Give students a piece of paper with each letter of the alphabet printed on it and tell them that you are going to conduct an alphabet scavenger hunt. There will be several rounds, and you will give instructions for each 2-minute round.

Round 1: Students must find one item that starts with each letter of the alphabet. During round one, which lasts 2 minutes, they can write down only those things they personally have (on their person, in backpack, purse, etc.).

Round 2: Students may join with one other person to combine efforts, still using only what one or the other has on him- or herself (or in backpack, purse, etc.).

Round 3: Each pair may combine with one other pair to combine lists. (Two more minutes are allowed.)

Continue adding students to the group each round. The number of rounds will change depending on how many students are involved in the activity. After completing the lists as much as possible, use the following questions to discuss with group members what they noticed during the activity:

- Did it get easier to add to the list as time went on?
- How does the point of this exercise apply in life during times of stress or difficulty?
- Why is it important to have more than one or two people in your support group?

LINKED ELBOW STAND (ALL AGES)

Have two students sit back to back, linking elbows. Instruct them that they are to stand up at the same time without unlinking elbows. In order to stand at the same time, students must lean against each other while pushing up. After students have successfully stood up, discuss how leaning on another was needed in order to stand. Apply the activity to their lives.

Communication Activities

COMMUNICATION TENNIS (AGES 6 AND OLDER)

Explain to students that conversation is like playing a game of tennis (while talking, hold up a picture of a tennis player or tennis racket) and that the game has rules. Both players must start the game in their stance with their rackets ready to hit the ball (conversation) back and forth. Here are some basic communication skills to practice with student:

1. Ask, "Is it a good time to talk?" Ask this question directly. If it is not a good time, write a note, talk with another person, or wait until later.
2. Look at the other person while talking and do not speak too loudly or too softly.
3. Ask a question.
4. Wait for the other person's answer.
5. Keep the conversation going back and forth; conversation is similar to tennis players hitting a tennis ball back and forth on a tennis court.

Give the following directions (allow 2½ minutes to practice communication skills): "Pair up and practice a conversation. Talk about what we discussed today. Begin by asking, 'Is this a good time to talk?' The conversation should go back and forth between you, like the tennis ball in a game of tennis."

EYE CONTACT BALL GAME (AGES 6 AND OLDER)

Gather students in a circle. Pair each student with someone on the opposite side of the circle. Explain: "The goal is to throw the foam ball back and forth as each pair tries to keep up a conversation. Look at your partner and try to keep the conversation going. After the speaking partner ends a sentence or comment, he or she will throw the ball to the listening partner. The person who is speaking should be holding the ball. Start slow and go faster, seeing how fast you and your partner can start and end sentences without dropping the ball."

Students may become frustrated, but remind them: "You must work together. Good communication requires patience. This game is like a conversation. Conversation requires give and take. Conversation requires two people to work together."

"I FEEL" MESSAGES (AGES 8 AND OLDER)

Invite students to share how they have used their good communication skills over the past week. Expand on the previously taught conversation skills by teaching them how to use "I feel" statements. Read the scenarios listed below (one at a time) and ask students how they would feel in that particular situation. Practice using the formula: "I feel _____ when _____ because _____." You can normalize their feelings by making a statement after the student's "I Feel" statement. Using the student's phrases, you would insert: "Lots of kids feel _____ when _____ because _____." Considering the age of students involved, you might use the following examples:

- "Your dog chewed your new pair of shoes."
- "You were selected to be the class president."
- "Your mother is taking you to a restaurant for dinner tonight."
- "You earned a good grade on the math test."
- "Your best friend got sick and can't spend the night at your house."
- "You hit a home run for your baseball team."
- "You are late for school because your ride did not come on time.

Problem-Solving Activities

TANGLED ARMS GAME (ALL AGES)

Have students stand in a tight circle, facing inward with their eyes closed. Ask them to reach into the middle of the circle and grab the hand of someone else. Each student grabs another student's hand, preferably not the hand of a student standing next to him or her in the circle. Everyone opens their eyes. Students arms will be in a tangled mass. Ask students to work together to untangle their arms without letting go of each others' hands. The grip can be adjusted but not released. Students can almost always untangle their arms, but they may need encouragement. After all arms have been untangled, students will be standing in a circle with some children facing toward the center of the circle and some facing away from the center. Praise them for their perseverance.

PROBLEM SOLVING (AGES 8 AND OLDER)

Discuss how students were able to untangle their twisted arms and hand out Worksheet 5.8 for the following activity. (You can also use Overhead 5.8.) Explain that the following steps can help students solve almost any problem:

1. Define the problem.
2. Is it your problem? If not, whose is it?
3. Brainstorm possible solutions. When students are brainstorming, they don't stop to judge the ideas. It is important to list as many ideas as possible.
4. Look at each idea and ask "How would this solution work?"

5. Choose the best solution for the problem. This is personal. What might work well for one student might not work for another. Students need to evaluate their own situation and determine which solution will best fit their needs and circumstances.

6. Act on the chosen solution. Do it.

7. Review: Was the problem solved? If the problem is solved, GOOD JOB! If not, go back and try again.

Ask students to pick a problem that the whole group could use as an example. Use this example to demonstrate the seven steps of problem solving. Ask students to use the worksheet while practicing problem-solving skills with the example chosen by the group.

Self-Image Activity

AROUND THE TABLE COMPLIMENTS (AGES 8 AND OLDER)

Tell students: "Today we are going to learn about some things we can do to feel good about ourselsves. We are also going to talk about giving compliments and using descriptive words." Ask: "What is a compliment? When/why do you give compliments? How do you give compliments? What makes a good compliment?"

Instructions: "Today, we are going to give each other compliments. Because of time, we need to shorten the compliment to just one word. The word we are going to use is called an adjective. What is an adjective? Let's list some positive adjectives on the board." (Brainstorm a list of several possibilities.)

Pass out index cards and instruct students to write their name at the top of the card. To begin, they are to write a positive adjective about themselves at the very beginning. After 5–10 seconds, tell students to pass their card to the next person. The only rule about what they can write is that it has to be positive. Tell students that if the adjective is already there, they cannot write it again. It may also be a good idea to talk about what they should do if they do not really know the person or if they do not like the person.

At the end of the activity, give students a minute or two to look over their cards, then begin the discussion.

Possible discussion questions:

- "After you've read the things on the card, what are you thinking about?"
- "Some people find it difficult to read nice things about themselves, whereas others find it easier. Why do you think that is?"
- "What is *self-image*?"
- "What does it mean to have a positive self-image?"
- "What does it mean to have a negative self-image?"
- "What contributes to a positive self-image?"
- "Why might a person have a negative self-image?"
- "How can a person improve his or her self-image?"
- "What can you do this week to improve your self-image? Write a goal on the card."

Possible alternative: Another way this can be done that is also fun is called a "snow-ball" fight. Each student has a piece of paper that they wrinkle up into a ball. They throw the ball into the center of the room. On the signal, everyone grabs a piece of paper, unwrinkles it and writes something nice about the person whose paper it is. They re-crinkle it and throw it back to the center then get another paper. This works well for a smaller class in which students can remember how many they have written on. The paper does get a little soft and is easier to tear, but the kids have fun with it.

Possible follow-up: After the discussion, have students choose the three of their qualities. Give each student three colored strips of paper. Have them write the qualities on the strip of paper with their initials. Then make a paper chain with each students qualities to hang in front of the classroom. (This could also be done as a school-wide activity, having teachers hang the chain outside on the wall . . . see if you can make a chain that goes around the whole school).

SUGGESTED READING

Albano, A., & Kendall, P. (2002). Cognitive behavioural therapy for children and adolescents with anxiety disorders: Clinical research advances. *International Review of Psychiatry, 14,* 129–134.

Brandon, R. (2003). *Family matters: Mental health of children and parents.* Policy brief. Washington University, Seattle. Human Services Policy Center (ED 478231)

Criss, M., Pettit, G., Bates, J., Dodge, K., & Lapp, A. (2002). Family adversity, positive peer relationships, and children's externalizing behavior: A longitudinal perspective on risk and resilience. *Child Development, 73*(4), 1220–1237.

Cunningham, N., & Sandhu, D. (2000). A comprehensive approach to school–community violence prevention. *Professional School Counseling, 4*(2), 126–133.

Doll, B., Zucker, S., & Brehm, K. (2004). *Resilient classrooms: Creating healthy environments for learning.* New York: Guilford Press.

Elliot, S., Kratochwill, T., & Roach, A. (2003). Commentary: Implementing social–emotional and academic innovations: Reflections, reactions, and research. *School Psychology Review, 32*(3), 320–327.

Frydenberg, E., & Lewis, R. (1999). The adolescent coping scale: Construct validity and what the instrument tells us. *Australian Journal of Guidance Counseling, 9,* 19–36.

Frydenberg, E., & Lewis, R. (2002). Adolescent well-being: Building young people's resources. In E. Frydenberg (Ed.), *Beyond coping: Meetings goals, vision and challenges* (175–194). Oxford, UK: Oxford University Press.

Frydenberg, E. (2004). Coping competencies: What to teach and when. *Theory into Practice, 43*(1), 14–21.

Gaylord, N., Kitzmann, K., & Lockwood, R. (2003). Child characteristics as moderators of the association between family stress and children's internalizing, externalizing, and peer rejection. *Journal of Child and Family Studies, 12*(2), 201–213.

Hoagwood, K., & Erwin, H. (1997). Effectiveness of school-based mental health services for children: A 10-year research review. *Journal of Child and Family Studies, 6*(4), 435–451.

Howard, S., & Johnson, B. (2000). What makes the difference? Children and teachers talk about resilient outcomes for children "at risk." *Educational Studies, 26*(3), 321–337.

Klicker, R. L. (1999). *A student dies, a school mourns: Dealing with death and loss in the school community*. Ann Arbor, MI: Taylor & Francis.

Lightfoot, J., Wright, S., & Sloper, P. (1999). Supporting pupils in mainstream school with an illness or disability: Young people's views. *Child: Care, Health and Development, 25*(4), 267–283.

Maleki, C., & Elliot, S. (2002). Children's social behaviors as predictors of academic achievement: A longitudinal analysis. *School Psychology Quarterly, 17*, 1–23.

Monahon, C. (1997). *Children and trauma: A guide for parents and professionals*. San Francisco: Jossey-Bass.

Percy, M., (2003). Feeling loved, having friends to count on, and taking care of yourself: Minority children living in poverty describe what is "special" to them. *Journal of Children and Poverty, 9*(1), 55–70.

Richardson, C. D., & Rosen, L. A. (1999). School-based interventions for children of divorce. *Professional School Counseling, 3*, 21–26.

Shaw, J. (2000). Children, adolescents and trauma. *Psychiatric Quarterly, 71*(3), 227–243.

Staudt, M. (2001). Psychopathology, peer relations, and school functioning of maltreated children: A literature review. *Children and Schools, 23*(2), 85–101.

UCLA School Mental Health Project. Online at *smhp.psych.ucla.edu/*

Velting, O., Setzer, N., & Albano, A. (2004). Update on and advances in assessment and cognitive-behavioral treatment of anxiety disorders in children and adolescents. *Professional Psychology, Research and Practice, 35*(1), 42–54.

Thoughts Connect with Feelings (Ages 8 and Older)

Name: _____

For the five pictures in the left column, describe a thought under the smiling face about each picture that might make someone feel happy, and describe a thought under the frowning face that might make someone feel sad.

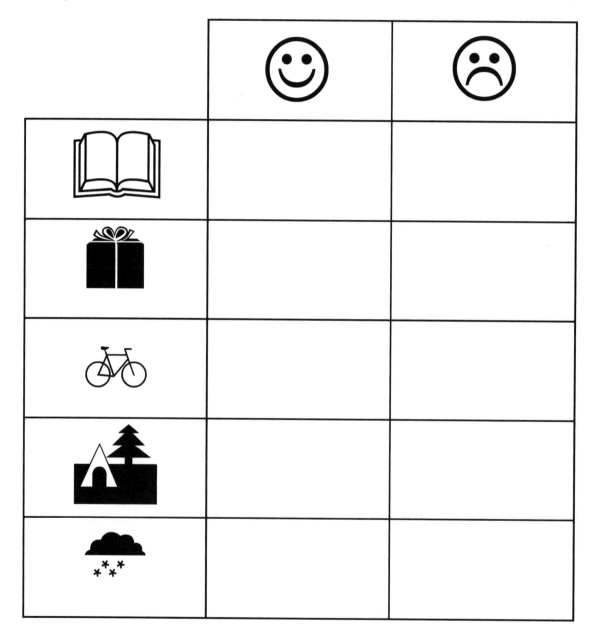

We Aren't "Bugged"! (Teacher Copy)

Bugs teach us many things about dealing with hard situations. Write an interesting fact about each bug and what we learn from the bug's example.

The bug	Interesting fact	What do we learn?
Dung Beetle	Dung beetles push dung into little balls. They eat it as well as use it to build their homes.	They make the best of stinky situations. We can also make the best of our stinky situations. Hard situations help us grow.
Flea	Fleas can jump a foot high, but they can't fly.	Even though they can't fly like other insects, fleas use the skills they have. We each have different skills from others. We can't do everything, but we can use the skills we have.
Termite	Termites can't survive alone. Every termite contributes to the community. Even blind termites are workers. Blind termites keep the termites' home in good repair. They also find food for other termites to eat.	EVERYONE has something they can contribute. We need to be OK with letting others help us.
Bees	Bees cooperate with each other to make honey.	When difficult things happen, we can work together to find solutions.
Dragonfly	Dragonflies are the fastest insects in the world. They have four wings and can hover like a helicopter. They can fly backward. They can change direction in mid-flight without stopping.	Sometimes we are comfortable with one way of doing something. But it is important to change direction if we need to. If we are trying to do something that isn't working, we need to change direction and try something different.
Wasp	Wasps have a "wasp waist." Their waist is connected to the rest of their body by a tiny joint. This joint makes it easy for them to move around in very cramped spaces.	Just like a wasp getting around in cramped spaces, being flexible makes it easier for us to get through difficult situations.

We Aren't "Bugged"!

Name: _____

Bugs teach us many things about dealing with hard situations. Write an interesting fact about each bug and what we learn from the bug's example.

The bug	Interesting fact	What do we learn?
Dung Beetle		
Flea		
Termite		
Bees		
Dragonfly		
Wasp		

Divorce Worksheet (Ages 8–12)

Fill in the blanks using the words below.

(a) messages   (b) parents   (c) directly   (d) alone

(e) changes   (f) married   (g) beginning   (h) nothing

Sometimes parents get divorced. But they are still our _____.

The word *divorced* means no longer _____.

Sometimes parents change how they feel about each other. There is _____ kids can do to stop this.

Divorce brings many _____ to the family. Some changes seem bad, others not so bad, and some are good.

It's not a kid's job to send _____ from one parent to the other. Parents need to talk _____ to each other.

Divorce can be hard to accept. But remember, it can also be the _____ of a new life.

Many kids have divorced parents. You are not _____.

Key: b, f, h, e, a, c, g, d

Feelings about Divorce (Ages 6–12)

Kids can't control how their parents feel or act. Parents get married for grown-up reasons, and they get divorced for grown-up reasons. Kids don't cause divorce. They can't stop divorce. But everyone has feelings about it.

Draw some pictures in these boxes to show how kids feel about their parents' divorce.

Masks (Ages 5–11)

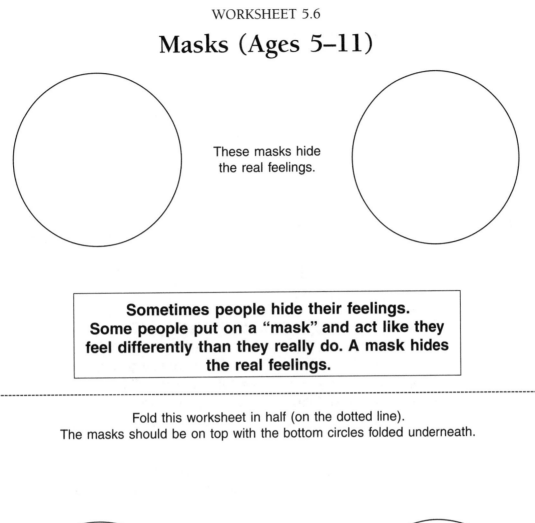

These masks hide
the real feelings.

Sometimes people hide their feelings.
Some people put on a "mask" and act like they
feel differently than they really do. A mask hides
the real feelings.

Fold this worksheet in half (on the dotted line).
The masks should be on top with the bottom circles folded underneath.

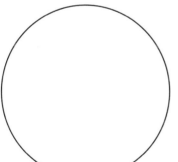

These are
the real feelings.

Masks (Ages 12–18)

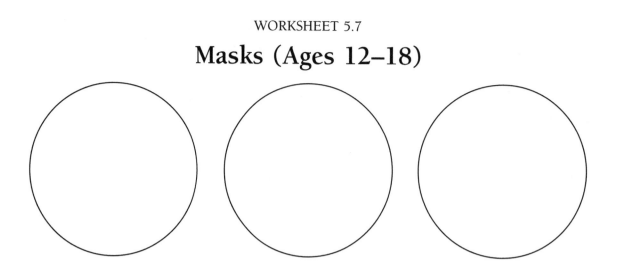

These masks hide the real feelings.

> **Sometimes people hide their feelings. They might worry that their feelings are not normal. Others might wonder if it is OK to have these feelings. Some people put on a "mask" by pretending to feel differently than they really do. A mask hides the real feelings.**

Fold this worksheet in half (on the dotted line).
The masks should be on top with the bottom circles folded underneath.

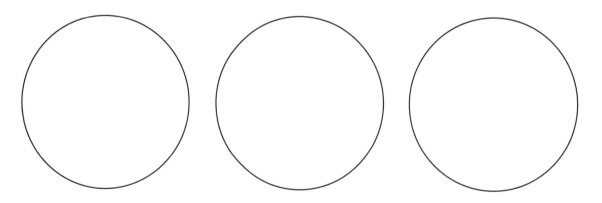

The bottom circles represent real feelings that the masks are hiding.

Problem-Solving Steps (Ages 8 and Older)

Name: _____

	Define the problem.
	Is it your problem? If not, whose is it?
	Brainstorm possible solutions. Don't stop to judge ideas, just list any idea you think of.
	Look at each idea and ask "How would this solution work?"
	Choose the best solution for the problem.
	Act on your solution.
	Review: Was the problem solved? If so, GOOD JOB! If not, go back and try again.

Topic: Depression

Depression is a state of sadness that lasts for long periods of time. When a child is grieving about something, sadness is common. If the sadness lasts for a long time or interferes a great deal with everyday functioning, it may be depression.

Causes of depression

Many things may cause depression. The condition may be related to a chemical imbalance in the brain, stress at home or school, the death of loved ones, self-esteem issues, or the student's perception about how much he or she controls what happens in his or her life. Regardless of the cause, depressed students tend to struggle more academically.

Signs of depression

The signs of depression vary depending on the individual and developmental levels. Some basic things to look for include:

- Irritability
- Nervousness
- Apathy
- Withdrawal
- Feelings of worthlessness
- Feelings of hopelessness
- Decreased concentration
- Crying often
- Acting out
- Change in eating habits
- Losing or gaining weight
- Physical complaints
- Inability to sleep or sleeping too much
- Self-injury
- Discussion of, or attempt of, suicide

What to do when a student seems depressed

- Be aware of how student's mood affects academic performance.
- Pay attention to student reactions to self; help him or her speak positively to self about self.
- Help student feel loved and accepted.
- Take time to listen to student
- Say, "I notice . . ." to student about specific things (not necessarily behaviors) each day.
- Seat student near an accepting peer.
- Empower student by providing choices when possible.
- If behavior is unacceptable, respond accordingly, reacting to the behavior, *not* the student.
- Be consistent in classroom discipline.
- Be alert to possible suicidal intentions and get help immediately.
- Contact parents about concerns.
- Refer to school mental health professional, if needed.

Topic: Chronic and Serious Illness

Students with chronic and serious illness struggle with a variety of issues in a school setting. Chronic absences, limited participation in school activities, teacher response to students' struggles, and peer relationships all influence the overall well-being of students with chronic illness. There is much a teacher can watch for and do to accommodate these students and help them feel successful as they grapple with managing their illness while at school.

Specific struggles of students with chronic illness

- Absenteeism resulting in difficulties with schoolwork and consistent peer relationships
- Feeling out of place, different or isolated
- Being bullied
- Being disregarded
- Dealing with side-effects of medications
- Coping with pain and fatigue
- Trouble with motor coordination

What teachers can do

- Become aware of implications of illness for student at school.
- Ask student what he or she needs.
- Take time to explain missing assignments.
- Be flexible with deadlines.
- Empower student to make decisions about his or her education.
- Adapt activities requiring physical exertion.
- Pay attention to bullying situations and take appropriate action.
- Be careful what is mentioned about (or to) student in front of peers.
- Encourage peer relationships by including friends in the accommodations.
- Teach and encourage tolerance for diversity.

Students who are chronically ill may require extra attention and care in an educational setting. As teachers take time to be aware of individual situations, they will be more prepared to assist. Children need to feel important and included in group settings. Positive peer relationships are essential to students' support networks. It is helpful when teachers take action to assist students in building relationships by eliminating stigma and increasing tolerance for diversity. Chronic illness is a condition the student must deal with; it is not who the student is. Becoming sensitive and responsive to the special needs of students with chronic illness is essential.

RESOURCES:

Lightfoot, J., Wright, S., & Sloper, P. (1999). Supporting pupils in mainstream school with an illness or disability: Young people's views. *Child: Care, Health and Development, 25*(4), 267–283.
Steward, M. S. (2002). Illness: A crisis for children. In J. Sandoval (Ed.), *Handbook of crisis counseling, intervention, and prevention in the schools* (2nd ed., pp. 183–211). Mahwah, NJ: Erlbaum.

Topic: Difficulties Making and Keeping Friends

Parents, teachers, and friends all play a significant role in children's development. Friends, in particular, are important to children. Unfortunately, many children struggle with making and keeping friends.

Positive friendships provide:

- Emotional support
- Help with problems
- Differing points of view
- Positive social experiences
- Opportunities to learn and practice social skills
- Opportunities to practice empathy

Children without friends:

- Feel lonely
- Are more likely to be bullied by peers
- Have lower self-esteem
- Have difficulties adjusting to school
- Exhibit problem behaviors
- Are at higher risk for depression or other mental health problems

Students who struggle with peer relationships may be bossy, impulsive, or unkind. They may appear judgmental of peers and insult others. Students who do not interact well with peers may also be withdrawn and not recognize or respond to attempts at friendship. Overall, difficulty making and keeping friends seems to be rooted in poor social skills.

Examples of needed social skills:

- Cooperation
- Communication
- Greeting others
- Making requests
- Listening

- Maintaining eye contact
- Conveying empathy and tact
- Receiving feedback
- Responding to peer rejection
- Compromising

What you can do:

Students without friends often need to be taught how to make friends. Teachers can observe those who struggle to determine what skills the students need to learn. They can then teach and encourage individual students to use necessary skills with their peers in everyday interactions.

RESOURCES:

Children without Friends National Network for Child Care. *Children without friends*. Available online at *www.nncc.org/Guidance/dc26_wo.friends1.html*

Topic: Divorce

Approximately half of all marriages end in divorce (Amato, 2001). Because divorce is so common, it is important to support students affected by it. In order to assist students, school personnel can increase their understanding of how students are affected by divorce.

DIFFICULTIES FACED BY CHILDREN

Divorce is complicated and difficult for children and adolescents to understand. They are often confused about why parents divorce. Children wonder where they fit into the restructured family. Frequently, they blame themselves for the divorce. Although children have many concerns and questions, they are hesitant to ask their parents about the divorce. Lacking information, they hold on to misconceptions and fears related to divorce. They feel alone.

BUILDING RESILIENCE

Current divorce literature provides information on key issues related to children's adjustment in family transitions and how to provide appropriate support. The research findings are optimistic in regard to children's adaptability and resilience (Hetherington & Stanley-Hagan, 1999). For children experiencing parental divorce, positive outcomes are strongly correlated with availability of emotionally responsive adults and parents who provide a strong basis of emotional support (Amato, 2001).

RESILIENCE SKILLS

Most students benefit from learning and practicing the following skills:

- Expressing feelings in appropriate ways
- Solving problems
- Developing and strengthening friendships

Topic: Abuse

Physical: Physical injury inflicted on a child

- Includes bruises, scrape, or abrasions

Sexual: Any sexual contact between a child and an adult or older child

- Manipulation, force, and threats are used.
- Contact ranges from inappropriate touching to sodomy or intercourse.

Emotional: Using actions or words that demean or degrade a child

- Includes verbal insults, name calling, screaming, negative comparisons with others, and other acts that cause shame

SIGNS OF ABUSE

Physical

- Bruises in shapes that that look like handprints or objects
- Black eyes
- Broken bones
- Injuries after being absent
- Pattern of injuries without sufficient explanation
- Poor medical or dental care
- Inappropriate hygiene
- Constant hunger or thirst
- Unexplained physical complaints

Behavioral

- Unexpected change in behavior
- Behavior typical of someone younger
- Cringing or shying away when approached by someone
- Frequent blank stares/spacing out
- Poor sleep or frequent nightmares
- Irrational fears
- Excessive fear of a specific person
- Acting out sexually

IT IS REQUIRED BY LAW TO REPORT ALL <u>SUSPECTED</u> ABUSE TO THE AUTHORITIES!

- Report facts as facts and suspicion as suspicion.
- You do not have to prove there is abuse—that is what the authorities do.
- You are not required to tell parents about report if they are suspected abusers.

Topic: Abuse

Teachers and staff are required to report all *suspected* abuse to the proper authorities, typically Child Protective Services or the Department of Human Services. If you suspect abuse, report it. Clearly report the facts as facts and suspicion as suspicion. If you do not know which phone number to call, ask your principal, school nurse, or mental health professional. There are also national hotlines open for calls 24 hours a day. Toll-free hotline numbers are listed in phone books. Most schools have an outlined routine for reporting suspected abuse. Some schools may want you to file a short written report with the school nurse or principal. Find out what your school policy is and follow the guidelines.

Remember, you do not have to prove that there was abuse. Your duty is to report suspected abuse, then let the authorities investigate the claims. You are not required to inform the parents if they are the perpetrators of abuse. In fact, if they later ask you if you reported the suspected abuse, you can state: "Anyone in the school may have reported their concerns to the authorities. By law, all adults are required to report suspected abuse. So it may have been any adult in the school."

Although many cases of abuse are not life threatening, in extreme cases in which the student's safety is in question, let the principal, school counselor, or school psychologist know immediately. He or she can support you in getting proper help for the student. Do not take on the responsibility for solving the problem. This is not your responsibility.

In response to the abuse, children may feel guilt, shame, isolation, and fear. Feeling powerless, they may also feel hopeless and depressed. Some children may consider suicide or running away to escape the abuse; some may suffer with high levels of anxiety that render them easily startled and sensitive to loud noises or touch.

Teachers and staff should consult with mental health professionals to determine how to adapt their classroom to the needs of the student with a history of abuse. The goal is to reduce stress and anxiety, creating an environment in which the student feels safe and secure. Suggested interventions may be as simple as seating the student in the back corner of the classroom, he or she can see everything and feel more in control. Other students may feel more secure being seated next to the teacher's desk or near the door or window. Specific situations may require different strategies, depending on the student's worries and fears. In extreme cases of anxiety, the student may need a hall pass to visit with the school counselor.

Topic: Suicide

PROBLEMS THAT MAY PUT STUDENTS AT RISK:

Family Problems	Personal Problems	School Problems
Frequent moves	Alcoholism/drug abuse	Failing grades
Money problems	Abuse (physical, sexual, or emotional)	Learning disability
Marital conflict		Discipline problems
Separation or divorce	Breakup/fight with boyfriend/girlfriend	Peer rejection
Domestic violence	Mental illness	Harassment (bullying, sexual harassment)
Family history of suicide and/or depression	Depression	
Excessive discipline	Previous suicide attempts	
Too much or too little control/supervision	Legal problems/delinquency	
Serious or ongoing illness	Pregnancy	
Student feels parents do not care	Feelings of isolation	
Parent–child conflicts/fights		
Death in family		

What should you do if a student is thinking about committing suicide?

1. **Listen**—Always listen to the student and let him or her know that you care.
   Be calm—The student will feel more secure and safe with adults who do not overreact.
   Remember—You can listen and be supportive; however, you are not the therapist. You do not counsel the student.
2. **Report concerns** to your supervisor or school counselor.
   Don't keep it a secret, even though the student may ask you not to tell.
   Tell student: "I care about you and want to get someone to help us. When you care about a person, you don't want him or her to hurt him- or herself. I want to help you."

What should you do if a student is talking about suicide or hurting him- or herself?

<u>Immediately</u> tell your supervisor and the school's mental health professional. If your school has a crisis plan, follow that plan for this type of situation. The school's mental health professional will talk with the student and determine what needs to be done. Do not leave a student alone if he or she is suicidal. Do not let the student use the restroom unattended.

Topic: Death and Grief

STAGES OF MOURNING

Sadness: Sadness is a common reaction to loss. Children may withdraw or show less interest in activities they previously enjoyed. Over time, the initial sadness should decrease as the child moves into other stages of grieving.

Denial: In response to loss, children may experience denial for several reasons. First, it is difficult to accept that a loved one is not coming back. Additionally, many unpleasant emotions accompany death. Difficulty tolerating intense emotion causes children to move into a fantasy world where they do not have to deal with death. This reaction is OK; however, if the child does not come back to reality, problems may result. Talking to the child about the person who died and recalling positive, loving, and happy experiences with him or her is helpful.

Guilt: Children may think that the death is their fault, or that they could have prevented it. Adults can remove this misperceived responsibility by repeatedly reassuring the child that the death was not their fault and that there is nothing they could have done to stop it.

Anger: The root of anger is often chaotic emotion that needs to be understood and expressed. Any change in life brings uncomfortable feelings. Emotions related to loss can be particularly confusing. Acting out that confusion via disruptive behavior is common. Adults can help by understanding where the anger comes from and having patience. Coaching the child in recognizing and expressing each emotion is also helpful.

Shame/Stigma: Children want to believe that they are like everyone else, that they blend into the crowd. When a loved one dies, it sets them apart as different. They may also feel embarrassed by the attention of adults paying condolences. When they experience a loss, they may feel different. Being different feels shameful. Involving a child with a group of peers who has experienced similar losses may be helpful.

Acceptance: As children who have experienced loss reach different stages in their development, they will recycle through the first steps of mourning. Children go through many milestones during which the missing presence of a loved one is noticed. Typically, children come to gradually accept death but continue to remember their loss, even into adulthood.

When speaking to a mourning student:
- Acknowledge the loss.
- Be direct, sensitive, and authentic.
- Avoid asking questions to satisfy your own curiosity.
- Let the student know that you are there if he or she wants to talk (offer a listening ear).
- Let student reminisce when ready.

To support a mourning student:
- Find a way to commemorate deceased person's life (e.g., donating a book to the library in his or her memory).
- Teach other children how to respond when student returns.
- Help student readjust to classroom routine as soon as possible.
- Allow for moments when student needs to be alone to grieve.
- Be aware of days or times of year that may be more difficult (e.g., family-centered holidays).

Grief

> **Sometimes bad things happen to people, even kids. Sometimes we lose something or someone very important to us. Our heart hurts. This pain is called grief. The grief will not always hurt so much. Grief comes and goes, like the waves on a beach.**

The first wave surprises us.
No one wants to believe
this is really happening.

Then comes a wave of
anger, confusion, worry,
or pain. Sometimes
many feelings come splashing
in all at once.

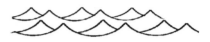

Talking about these
feelings helps you understand
them better. The waves will
calm you. Peace and healing will come
to your heart.

Just like the waves on the beach,
feelings are always there.
Sometimes they are upsetting and scary.
Other times they are peaceful and calm.
When the painful waves come back,
remember, you are not alone. Soon
the rough waves will calm and pass.

SEA GLASS

Metaphor: Sea Glass

Purpose: Putting painful feelings and memories into perspective; giving hope for the future.

Suggestion: Purchase sea glass from a craft store. Tell the story to a classroom of children. After telling the story, pass a piece of the sea glass around the classroom. Leave a piece of sea glass on the teacher's desk as a reminder of this story.

"Does anyone know what sea glass is? If you walk along an ocean shore, you will see sea glass. The ocean water and sand work together, gradually smoothing the sharp and jagged edges of broken glass. Over time, the glass becomes smooth and rounded on the edges. The glass is still there, but the edges no longer cut.

"Sometimes bad things happen. It makes our hearts sad. We hurt. We may be angry. These are strong feelings. You may wonder if they will ever go away. Broken glass is like your feelings. Right after the glass is broken, the sharp edges can cut and hurt you. Your feelings hurt. They feel sharp and jagged. Over time and with the support of others, the edges of your feelings become smooth and rounded. Even though the memory stays in your heart, it becomes softer. In the future, you will be able to think about what happened, and it won't hurt as much as it does right now."

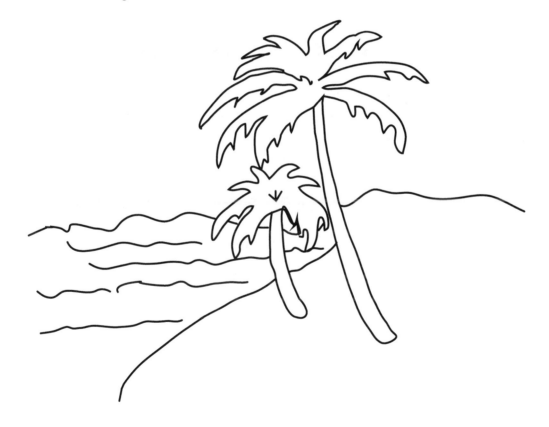

ABUSE: WHAT YOU CAN DO

> It is required BY LAW to report
> all **suspected** abuse to proper authorities

- Report facts as facts.

- Report suspicion as suspicion.

- You do not have to prove there is abuse—that is what the authorities do.

- You are not required to tell parents about report if they are suspected abusers.

CLASSROOM INTERVENTIONS

To meet individual needs, discuss possible interventions
with school counselor or school psychologist.

ABUSE

Physical: physical injury inflicted on a child

- Includes bruises, scrapes, or abrasions

Sexual: Any sexual contact between a child and an adult or older child

- Manipulation, force, and threats are used.
- Contact ranges from inappropriate touching to sodomy or intercourse.

Emotional: Using actions or words that demean or degrade a child

- Includes verbal insults, name calling, screaming, negative comparisons with others, and other acts that cause shame

Abuse causes: guilt, shame, isolation, fear, depression, hopelessness, helplessness

⚠ SIGNS OF ABUSE ⚠

Physical

- Bruises in shapes that look like handprints or objects
- Black eyes
- Broken bones
- Injuries after being absent
- Pattern of injuries without sufficient explanation
- Poor medical or dental care
- Inappropriate hygiene
- Constant hunger or thirst
- Unexplained physical complaints

Behavioral

- Unexpected change in behavior
- Behavior typical of someone younger
- Cringing or shying away when approached by someone
- Frequent blank stares/spacing out
- Poor sleep or frequent nightmares
- Irrational fears
- Excessive fear of a specific person
- Acting out sexually

CRYING FOR HELP

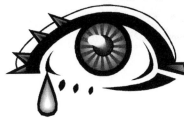

SIGNS OF SUICIDE

Problems adjusting
Lack of social connections
Extreme shame, anxiety, or depression
Alcohol or drug use
Sudden change in personality
Engaging in dangerous activities

History of suicidal behavior
Expressing suicidal plans
Loss of interest in life
Preoccupation with death
Preparation for death (giving away
    possessions)

**Report concerns to your supervisor
or school mental health professional immediately.**

IF A STUDENT IS THINKING ABOUT SUICIDE

Listen

Be calm

Tell student you care

Immediately report concerns

"When you care about a person, you don't want him or her to hurt him- or herself. I care about you and want to get someone to help. I want to help you."

THE MOURNING PROCESS

When a child experiences loss, the resulting feelings may be puzzling. There are several feelings that make up the mourning process.

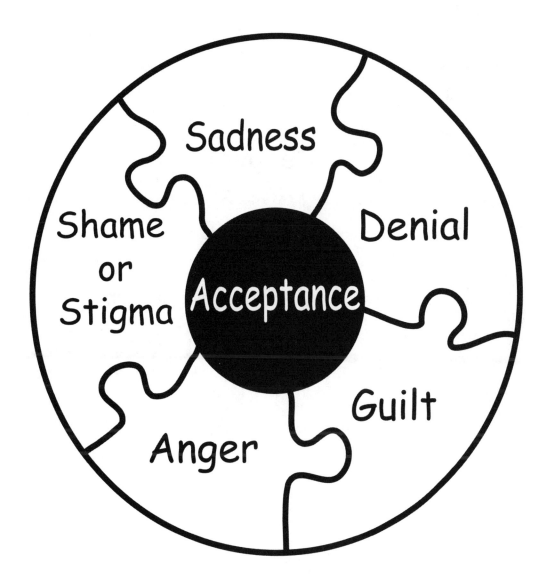

From Melissa Allen Heath and Dawn Sheen (2005). Copyright by The Guilford Press. Permission to photocopy this material is granted to purchasers of this book for personal use only (see copyright page for details).

DEFINING GROUP RULES

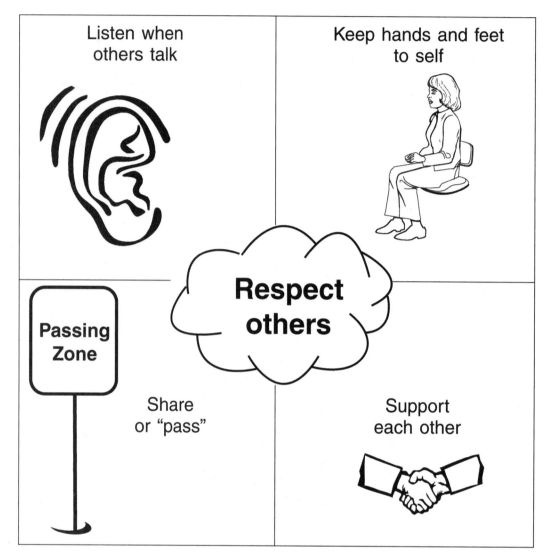

Listen when others talk

Keep hands and feet to self

Passing Zone

Respect others

Share or "pass"

Support each other

PROBLEM-SOLVING STEPS

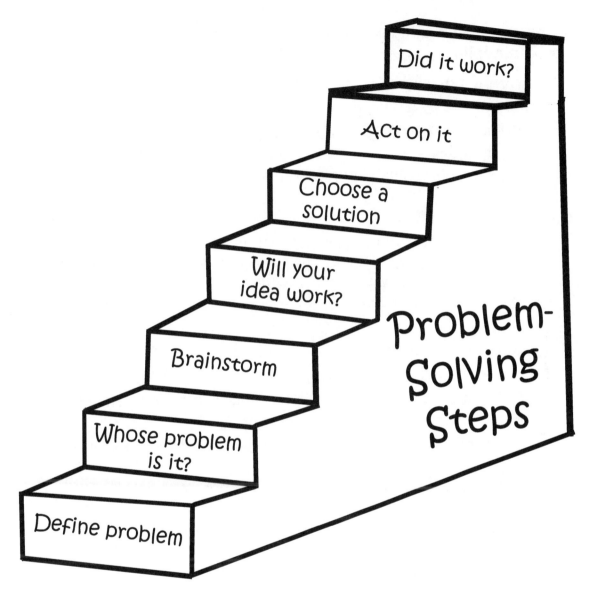

ANXIETY

When faced with difficulty or a threat, anxious students go on autopilot:

(1) SURVIVAL MODE

THOUGHT: It's me against the world.
RESPONSE: *FIGHT,* DEFEND SELF
FEELINGS: ANGER
Note: Reaction seems extreme in relation to the threat.

(2) SURRENDER MODE

THOUGHT: I can't. I am hopeless and helpless.
RESPONSE: *FLIGHT*, ESCAPE PROBLEM, RUN FROM PROBLEM,
    TUNE OUT, or GIVE UP
FEELINGS: FEAR, TERROR

Suggestions for teachers:

1. Teach relaxation skills to entire class.
2. Foster a safe classroom climate: no bullying or harassment.
3. Reduce noise level of classroom.
4. Teach and encourage problem-solving strategies and skills.

BIBLIOTHERAPY SUMMARY 5.1

Book Title	When Addie Was Scared		Excellent	Fair	Poor
Issue Addressed	Fear/anxiety	Developmental Level	X		
Author(s)	Linda Bailey	Language and Writing Style	X		
Year of Publication	1999	Quality of Illustrations	X		
Publisher	Kids Can Press	Life Experiences	X		
Address of Publisher		Portrayal of Problems	X		
ISBN #	1-55074-431-3	Problem-Solving Process	X		
Price	$14.95	Coping Skills	X		
Age/Grade Level	K–grade 3	Characterization	X		
# of Pages	Approx. 32	Dialogue and Communication Skills	X		
Summary of Story: Addie is scared of everything, until one day she finds the courage inside herself to face one of her fears.		Purpose of Emotionally Charged Scenes	X		
		Sensitivity to Human Diversity	X		
		Hope and Support	X		

Suggested Activity

Have students draw a picture of their greatest fear. Then have them draw a picture of themselves bigger than their fear. Discuss why they can be bigger than their fear, pointing out actions they can take to be less afraid.

BIBLIOTHERAPY SUMMARY 5.2

Book Title	Joey Pigza Swallowed the Key		Excellent	Fair	Poor
Issue Addressed	Anxiety, ADHD	Developmental Level	X		
Author(s)	Jack Gantos	Language and Writing Style	X		
Year of Publication	1998	Quality of Illustrations	NA		
Publisher	Farrar, Straus & Giroux	Life Experiences	X		
Address of Publisher	New York	Portrayal of Problems	X		
ISBN #	0-37433-664-4	Problem-Solving Process	X		
Price	$5.99	Coping Skills	X		
Age/Grade Level	Grades 4–6	Characterization	X		
# of Pages	154	Dialogue and Communication Skills	X		
Summary of Story: Joey Pigza can't sit still. He struggles at school and at home. He worries a lot about behaving better but doesn't know how to slow down. When his behavior gets out of hand at school, more drastic measures are taken to help him.		Purpose of Emotionally Charged Scenes	X		
		Sensitivity to Human Diversity	X		
		Hope and Support	X		

Suggested Activity

Joey Pigza struggled with making good decisions. Teach students about decision making and problem solving using Tangled Arms Game (p. 100) and "Problem-Solving Steps" (Worksheet 5.8; see also "Additional Activities," pp. 90–91).

BIBLIOTHERAPY SUMMARY 5.3

			Excellent	Fair	Poor
Book Title	*How to Lose All Your Friends*				
Issue Addressed	*Friendship problems*	Developmental Level	X		
Author(s)	*Nancy Carlson*	Language and Writing Style	X		
Year of Publication	*1997*	Quality of Illustrations	X		
Publisher	*Puffin*	Life Experiences	X		
Address of Publisher	*New York*	Portrayal of Problems	X		
ISBN #	*0-14055-862-4*	Problem-Solving Process	X		
Price	*$5.99*	Coping Skills	X		
Age/Grade Level	*Pre-K–grade 2*	Characterization	X		
# of Pages	*Approx. 32*	Dialogue and Communication Skills	X		
Summary of Story: *A cute story with great pictures listing all the ways a person can lose his or her friends.*		Purpose of Emotionally Charged Scenes	X		
		Sensitivity to Human Diversity	X		
		Hope and Support	X		

Suggested Activity

After a class discussion, have students write and illustrate their own book about how to lose all their friends. OR, have students write and illustrate a book about how to keep all their friends.

BIBLIOTHERAPY SUMMARY 5.4

			Excellent	Fair	Poor
Book Title	When Zachary Beaver Came to Town				
Issue Addressed	Parent problems (separation), tolerance, obesity, neglect, death	Developmental Level	X		
Author(s)	Kimberly Willis Holt	Language and Writing Style	X		
Year of Publication	1999	Quality of Illustrations	NA		
Publisher	Henry Holt	Life Experiences	X		
Address of Publisher	New York	Portrayal of Problems	X		
ISBN #	0-80506-116-9	Problem-Solving Process	X		
Price	$16.95	Coping Skills	X		
Age/Grade Level	Grades 6–10	Characterization	X		
# of Pages	227	Dialogue and Communication Skills	X		
Summary of Story: The summer Toby's mother leaves is the summer Zachary Beaver, the fattest boy in the world, comes to town. Over several months, they become friends and Toby works through emotions related to his parents' separation.		Purpose of Emotionally Charged Scenes	X		
		Sensitivity to Human Diversity	X		
		Hope and Support	X		

Suggested Activity

Use the "Backpack Activity" (pp. 91–92). Have students choose a character in the book who was symbolically carrying something in his or her backpack. Do a "Four Corners" activity where each corner in the room represents one character. Students go to their character's corner and discuss with classmates what he or she was carrying in his or her backpack. How did he or she release feelings? Was it effective? After students have discussed responses, have them return to their seats and quickly share as a class what characters held in their backpacks. Have students think about what they might be carrying in their own backpack. Have them write a journal entry with a goal about how they can lighten their load.

BIBLIOTHERAPY SUMMARY 5.5

			Excellent	Fair	Poor
Book Title	*My Louisiana Sky*				
Issue Addressed	*Tolerance for diversity, parent problems, death, bullying, problem solving, conflict resolution*	Developmental Level	*X*		
Author(s)	*Kimberly Willis Holt*	Language and Writing Style	*X*		
Year of Publication	*1998*	Quality of Illustrations	*X*		
Publisher	*Harry Holt*	Life Experiences	*X*		
Address of Publisher	*New York*	Portrayal of Problems	*X*		
ISBN #	*0-80505-251-8*	Problem-Solving Process	*X*		
Price	*$15.95*	Coping Skills	*X*		
Age/Grade Level	*Middle-high school*	Characterization	*X*		
# of Pages	*200*	Dialogue and Communication Skills	*X*		
Summary of Story: *Set in the 1950s, Tiger Ann has grown up with her grandmother and mentally slow parents. When her grandmother dies, she is faced with the decision of whether to live with her upper-class aunt in Baton Rouge or remain with her parents.*		Purpose of Emotionally Charged Scenes	*X*		
		Sensitivity to Human Diversity	*X*		
		Hope and Support	*X*		

Suggested Activity

Tiger Ann had many decisions to make. List some of the decisions she faced. What did she choose to do and why? Have students consider if they would have chosen differently. Why or why not? Form a values line as a class (in front of the classroom). One end of the line represents "Totally Agree," the other, "Totally Disagree." Students should stand in line in relation to how they felt about Tiger's decision. Fold the line in half so that Totally Agree and Totally Disagree are partners. Students discuss with partner what they think and why. After students sit down, have a quick class discussion. End by pointing out that although Tiger couldn't control many of the circumstances in her life (i.e., having mentally challenged parents), she could control the decisions she made about how to react. Assign students to write about how this idea applies in their lives.

BIBLIOTHERAPY SUMMARY 5.6

Book Title	Define "Normal"		Excellent	Fair	Poor
Issue Addressed	Parent mental illness, tolerance for differences	Developmental Level	X		
Author(s)	Julie Anne Peters	Language and Writing Style	X		
Year of Publication	2000	Quality of Illustrations	X		
Publisher	Little, Brown	Life Experiences	X		
Address of Publisher	New York	Portrayal of Problems	X		
ISBN #	0-31670-631-0	Problem-Solving Process	X		
Price	$5.99	Coping Skills	X		
Age/Grade Level	Middle school	Characterization	X		
# of Pages	Approx. 208	Dialogue and Communication Skills	X		
Summary of Story: This story describes the life of a student whose mother suffers from severe depression. The student gets involved in a peer counseling program in which the person with whom she is assigned to work seems completely beyond help. Throughout the process, the student finds she gains as much from her peer as she was hoping to give.		Purpose of Emotionally Charged Scenes	X		
		Sensitivity to Human Diversity	X		
		Hope and Support	X		

Suggested Activity

Write a journal entry about someone who is very different from you, yet from whom you learned an important lesson. Did you become friends? Explain how you developed a friendship with this person.

BIBLIOTHERAPY SUMMARY 5.7

			Excellent	Fair	Poor
Book Title	*Gettin' through Thursday*	Developmental Level	X		
Issue Addressed	*Financial difficulties*				
		Language and Writing Style	X		
Author(s)	*Melrose Cooper*				
		Quality of Illustrations	X		
Year of Publication	*1998*				
		Life Experiences	X		
Publisher	*Lee and Low Books*				
		Portrayal of Problems	X		
Address of Publisher	*New York*				
		Problem-Solving Process	X		
ISBN #	*1-88000-067-9*				
		Coping Skills	X		
Price	*$15.95*				
		Characterization	X		
Age/Grade Level	*Elementary*				
		Dialogue and Communication Skills	X		
# of Pages	*29*				
		Purpose of Emotionally Charged Scenes	X		
Summary of Story: *Thursdays are the hardest day for Andre's family. It's the day before payday when things start to run out. Usually it's OK, but one week, Andre is on the honor roll. Mama promised a party the day anyone got on the honor roll. But what happens when it falls on Thursday?*		Sensitivity to Human Diversity	X		
		Hope and Support	X		

Suggested Activity

Discuss what it feels like to want something but not be able to have it. Discuss Andre's feelings about not having the money to do what his mama promised. How was the problem resolved? What kinds of things can we have without spending money? In groups, have a contest to see who can write the most cost-free things for which they are thankful. Vocally compare lists. If two groups list the same item, they must cross it off. The group with the most original items wins. The last sentence in the book talks about a gift "that didn't cost a dime." What was that gift? How can we give the same type of gift to others? Have students brainstorm a list of things to do both at school and home, then choose one to act on during the next week.

BIBLIOTHERAPY SUMMARY 5.8

Book Title	Money Hungry		Excellent	Fair	Poor
Issue Addressed	Financial difficulties	Developmental Level	X		
Author(s)	Sharon Flake	Language and Writing Style		X	
Year of Publication	2001	Quality of Illustrations	NA		
Publisher	Hyperion Books for Children	Life Experiences	X		
Address of Publisher	New York	Portrayal of Problems	X		
ISBN #	0-78681-548-X	Problem-Solving Process		X	
Price	$5.99	Coping Skills		X	
Age/Grade Level	Middle school	Characterization	X		
# of Pages	187	Dialogue and Communication Skills	X		
Summary of Story: Raspberry Hill loves money. Ever since she and her mother have been off the streets, Raspberry does everything she can to earn money. She saves every penny in her bedroom, in hopes that she can help avoid being on the streets again.		Purpose of Emotionally Charged Scenes	X		
		Sensitivity to Human Diversity	X		
		Hope and Support	X		

Suggested Activity

Throughout the book, discuss the situation. Have students predict what will happen and discuss ending. Discuss characters' roles. Assign students to groups. Give groups a picture of a sun. Assign each group a different character's name to write in the circle in the middle. On the rays of the sun, list roles the character played. Have a spokesperson from each group share with class, then have class discuss character roles. Point out that everyone plays different roles in life. Some roles may be more difficult than others. In the roles we play, sometimes we take on more responsibility than necessary. It is important to recognize when we are playing a role that we don't need to play. Give students the picture with instructions to think about the roles they play, to be used for discussion later.

BIBLIOTHERAPY SUMMARY 5.9

			Excellent	Fair	Poor
Book Title	*Ramona and Her Father*				
Issue Addressed	*Financial difficulties*	Developmental Level	X		
Author(s)	*Beverly Cleary*	Language and Writing Style	X		
Year of Publication	*Reprint 1999*	Quality of Illustrations	X		
Publisher	*HarperTrophy*	Life Experiences	X		
Address of Publisher	*New York*	Portrayal of Problems	X		
ISBN #	*0-38070-916-3*	Problem-Solving Process	X		
Price	*$5.99*	Coping Skills	X		
Age/Grade Level	*Grades 2-4*	Characterization	X		
# of Pages	*180*	Dialogue and Communication Skills	X		
Summary of Story: *Ramona is in 2nd grade when her father loses his job. Story explores how Ramona wants to help as well as the worries she has related to the problem.*		Purpose of Emotionally Charged Scenes	X		
		Sensitivity to Human Diversity	X		
		Hope and Support	X		

Suggested Activity

Read book with students. Discuss Ramona's reaction to her father's losing his job. Could she really do anything to earn the money the family needed? How did she help? Brainstorm a list of things children <u>can</u> do to contribute to happier family environments when there's a lot of stress (e.g., helping more with household chores, getting along with siblings).

BIBLIOTHERAPY SUMMARY 5.10

			Excellent	Fair	Poor
Book Title	*Lilly's Purple Plastic Purse*				
Issue Addressed	*Conflict resolution*	Developmental Level	*X*		
Author(s)	*Kevin Henkes*	Language and Writing Style	*X*		
Year of Publication	*1996*	Quality of Illustrations		*X*	
Publisher	*Greenwillow Books*	Life Experiences		*X*	
Address of Publisher	*New York*	Portrayal of Problems	*X*		
ISBN #	*0-68812-897-1*	Problem-Solving Process	*X*		
Price	*$12.00*	Coping Skills	*X*		
Age/Grade Level	*4–9 years old*	Characterization	*X*		
# of Pages	*Approx. 32*	Dialogue and Communication Skills		*X*	
Summary of Story: *Lilly loves everything about school, until the day her teacher takes away her purple plastic purse. Story explores Lilly's reactions of sadness and anger. Also discusses how she reacts to the teacher and resolves the problem.*		Purpose of Emotionally Charged Scenes	*X*		
		Sensitivity to Human Diversity	*X*		
		Hope and Support	*X*		

Suggested Activity

Read book aloud, then discuss to ensure comprehension. Read a second time, asking students to pay attention to what Lilly does to fix the problem. Make a list of problem-solving steps. Give groups of students the same problem scenarios, asking them to use steps to find a solution. Discuss problems and solutions. Discuss how one problem can have many solutions. Ask students to rewrite the ending to *Lilly's Purple Plastic Purse* with a different solution.

BIBLIOTHERAPY SUMMARY 5.11

Book Title	*Is It Right to Fight?*			Excellent	Fair	Poor
Issue Addressed	*Anger*		Developmental Level	*X*		
Author(s)	*Pat Thomas*		Language and Writing Style	*X*		
Year of Publication	*2003*		Quality of Illustrations	*X*		
Publisher	*Barron's Educational Series*		Life Experiences	*X*		
Address of Publisher	*Hauppauge, NY*		Portrayal of Problems	*X*		
ISBN #	*0-76412-458-7*		Problem-Solving Process	*X*		
Price	*$5.95*		Coping Skills	*X*		
Age/Grade Level	*K–grade 4*		Characterization	*X*		
# of Pages	*Approx. 27*		Dialogue and Communication Skills	*X*		
Summary of Story: *Discusses different situations in which anger is an issue and fighting as a response to anger.*			Purpose of Emotionally Charged Scenes	*X*		
			Sensitivity to Human Diversity	*X*		
			Hope and Support	*X*		

Suggested Activity

With class, brainstorm what to do if someone is picking a fight. Role-play several scenarios in which fighting may be involved, assigning students to demonstrate alternate responses. In groups, students could also write skits in which anger is a problem. In their skits, they could write a desirable response and an undesirable response. Assign students to write about something that provokes anger in them and to include an action plan for how they will respond the next time it happens.

6

Preparing Noninstructional Personnel and Bus Drivers to Assist with Crisis Prevention and Intervention

MELISSA ALLEN HEATH *and* ELLIE L. YOUNG

NONINSTRUCTIONAL PERSONNEL

Noninstructional personnel include secretaries, office staff, bus drivers, custodial staff, and cafeteria workers. These individuals play a vital role in running a school. Indeed, they may be referred to as the "backbone of the school." With some basic training, these individuals can provide support during a school crisis or assist with critical incidents. On a day-to-day basis they can also provide emotional support to students. Additionally, noninstructional staff should be very familiar with the portions of the crisis plan that relate to their duties.

A secretary is typically the first person visitors see. Many times an angry parent vents his or her frustration on a secretary. The community depends on the secretary for a wide range of information. Often when the principal is out of the building, secretaries monitor misbehaving students in the office area until the principal returns. Therefore, secretaries and office aides, by default, end up handling a variety of student behavior problems. Secretaries also handle student mini crises such as forgotten lunches, lost items, desperate calls home, students who are late, scraped knees when the school nurse is unavailable, and so on. Given the multiple roles performed by school secretaries, basic training in listening

142

skills and behavior management would assist them in meeting the demands placed upon them.

The office staff assists with keeping records up to date and accurate. Parents' emergency contact numbers are critical during an emergency. The school may need to contact a parent or guardian in the case of student emergencies, such as when a student is injured or in need of immediate medical attention.

Communication during a crisis is critical. Parent, faculty, and staff phone trees are commonly part of a school crisis plan. However, outdated phone numbers are a common problem in emergency situations. Therefore, one critical responsibility of the office staff should be to keep all emergency contact numbers updated and to track down alternative numbers and e-mail addresses of parents and staff. Backup strategies for communication also need to be considered. For instance, your community might have an emergency radio or television station that broadcasts information regarding community or school procedures during an emergency. Another option to consider is keeping an emergency phone line in the school open specifically for emergencies. Whatever the plan, the school secretary and office staff must be familiar with the options for communicating during a school emergency. They must be able to direct parents and individuals from the community to an accurate information source.

PREPARING BUS DRIVERS TO ASSIST

Bus drivers play an important role in students' lives. Almost 25 million youth—half of all students in the United States—depend on school bus transportation to and from school (National School Transportation Association, 2002a). In regard to transporting students, a major concern of parents, bus drivers, and school administrators is students' physical safety. Based on accident reports, riding on the school bus is 2,000 times *safer* than riding in the family car (National School Transportation Association, 2002b). Of the approximately 800 student deaths occurring each year traveling to and from school, only 2% are associated with school bus accidents (*Education Week*, 2002). Those numbers support the notion that school buses are a safe mode of transportation.

However, even though school bus transportation is considered safe in terms of traffic accidents, other concerns arise in regard to student misbehavior. A bus driver has the responsibility of keeping control of both bus and student passengers. Considering that up to 72 students of varying ages are under the bus driver's charge, the task of maintaining order may seem overwhelming. Nevertheless, the bus driver is expected to manage student misbehavior and respond appropriately to crisis situations on the school bus.

The conditions on a school bus are a hotbed for student harassment and bullying. With limited adult supervision, inappropriate behaviors are much more likely to occur. Additionally, because the bus is separate from school, the driver may not feel connected with, or supported by, the school administrators. Interaction may be minimal. Because the bus driver has a difficult time communicating with the principal, who holds the disciplinary power over students, the driver may ignore minor misbehaviors. However, these minor infractions, such as sexual harassment or bullying, feed into more hostile and aggressive behaviors. Incidents of violence may reach the level of physical fights or worse: students bringing weapons to school for protection or retaliation.

Administrators must take several steps in assisting drivers to manage student behavior and prevent crisis situations on the school bus. It is important to provide an orientation for all new bus drivers, highlighting principles of managing student misbehavior. Invite the more seasoned bus drivers to assist with training. These drivers know the job and can give relevant practical examples, thereby grounding the training in reality. School administrators should attend a portion of the training to show their support, clarify responsibilities, review reporting procedures, and respond to questions.

In addition to defensive driving skills and information on bus care and maintenance, basic topics for training should include (1) procedures for reporting and assisting with accidents and accidental injuries; (2) bus evacuation procedures; (3) behavior management skills, particularly in dealing with bullying and sexual harassment; (4) reporting behavior problems to school authorities; and (5) strategies for conflict resolution and deescalation of student aggression and violence. All bus drivers should also be required to take a CPR and first aid class. At the very minimum, bus drivers must be able to provide immediate care when a student stops breathing, a student's heart stops beating, or in the case of severe bleeding. These three medical emergencies are life threatening and typically cannot wait for an ambulance or emergency care.

PREPARING CUSTODIAL STAFF AND CAFETERIA WORKERS TO ASSIST

Although custodial staff and cafeteria workers are not typically perceived as having authority over students or direct responsibility for students, they interact with students on an informal basis. Indeed, they are often aware of student problems that others may not have noticed.

Custodians are knowledgeable about the layout and physical characteristics of the school. They spend most of their time improving the school's physical environment for students and staff. They are aware of the building's features, which most students and teachers take for granted: alternative exit routes, location of electrical fuse boxes, gas lines, water lines, fire extinguishers, and ventilation ducts. They have master keys for the building. Custodians are an important group of individuals to include in planning and carrying out crisis intervention. They must be informed of the crisis plan and their role in it.

CONDUCTING STAFF TRAINING

Much of the training for bus drivers on crisis intervention overlaps with the training of other school staff. All staff who work with students, whether in the classroom or on the school bus, need a basic understanding of students' emotional needs. Understanding how to listen to students, particularly during crisis situations, is critical in providing crisis intervention. All school staff must be trained in providing emotional first aid to students in crisis.

All training for crisis intervention should include a review of the school discipline policy. School administrators are responsible for creating and implementing school policies, and school employees are responsible for upholding those policies. All employees should possess a copy of the school discipline policy and review it as part of training for crisis intervention. Those conducting the training should create role plays to demonstrate the policies that are most relevant to the group being trained.

The major focus of the training should be on preventing and managing student misbehavior, particularly bullying and sexual harassment. Staff must be told: "Do not ignore inappropriate behavior." All employees must be able to identify misbehavior. Rather than merely talking about it, role-play examples of misbehavior. Role plays provide an opportunity for participants to practice new skills. Following the role plays, the use of small group discussions can increase individual involvement and provide a less threatening forum for questions. It is also important to clarify expectations by role-playing specific examples of both appropriate and inappropriate responses. The following school bus scenario is followed by a role play. The role play clarifies what is expected of the bus driver when a student reports an incident of sexual harassment.

Scenario: You are a school bus driver. A ninth-grade female reports that two older boys on the bus flip her skirt up as she walks by their seat each day. She tells you this as she enters the school bus.

Discussion:

- What would you call this kind of behavior? (harassment/sexual harassment)
- How would you respond? (refer to school policy)

Role play: Choose two participants to role-play two different responses to this scenario.

Wrong response:

NINTH-GRADE FEMALE: Two boys are flipping my skirt up when I walk by them.

BUS DRIVER: If you wore pants, they wouldn't have a skirt to flip.

Correct response:

NINTH-GRADE FEMALE: Two boys are flipping my skirt up when I walk by them.

BUS DRIVER: Thank you for telling me. That's wrong for those boys to harass you. Please sit close to the front of the bus today. I'll talk with the boys about this and write a note to let the assistant principal know. Let me know if anything like this happens again.

Discussion:

- How does the first response differ from the second? Note: Sensitivity to students' feelings communicates respect and fosters a positive environment on the school bus. It is important to understand how difficult it is for students to report incidents of sexual harassment. When bus drivers ignore sexual harassment, students are less likely to report incidents, believing that "the bus driver won't do anything about it." It is important to stress that no student should experience sexual harassment under any circumstance.
- Refer to your school discipline plan. What is the school's policy on sexual harassment?
- If you were the bus driver, how would you report this behavior? Review the school's method for reporting and documenting incidents of sexual harassment. Review the following: when to report, to whom to report, and how to report. The situation must be reported particularly when students or parents complain.

Because they are not functioning in an instructional capacity, bus drivers, cafeteria workers, custodians, and secretaries depend on teachers and parents to teach students social skills and appropriate behaviors. Administrative support is vital in encouraging schoolwide prevention programs such as social skills curriculum or character education. All school employees, even those in noninstructional positions, should be familiar with the schoolwide prevention program. An overview of the program, with the basic information boiled down into a one-page handout, is helpful. They don't need to know all the details, but they do need to know basic information. They also need to be aware of information or policies that apply to their job and their association with students.

CRISIS INTERVENTION TOPICS FOR NONINSTRUCTIONAL STAFF

Many handouts for teachers can be modified for noninstructional staff. The training should involve basic skills. Short video clips and role plays are helpful in teaching listening skills (see Chapter 3). Overheads used for training teachers and instructional staff are also applicable. Training works best if at least part of the training is geared to a small group of staff holding similar positions. Small group discussions must be applicable to the specific group of employees. Employees will feel more comfortable in a discussion related to their employment and their experiences.

Providing each employee with a crisis plan is not sufficient. After formulating a tentative crisis plan, the proposed plan must be reviewed by those designated as responsible for various duties. Feedback should be solicited and used to make changes in the proposed plan. When staff members have a say in the crisis plan, they take ownership of their responsibilities and are much more likely to carry out their duties during a crisis.

Pertinent information from the crisis plan must be reviewed frequently in order to familiarize staff members with their duties. The plan should also be critiqued once a year to make changes, as needed. A representative from each group of school employees (secretarial, custodial, bus drivers, etc.) should participate in the yearly revision and updating of the crisis plan. At that time, key information related to each job should be discussed.

After a crisis situation, representatives should meet with their group and gather ideas on what went well during intervention and what aspects of the plan may need revision. The representative would then bring information back to the main crisis planning team and discuss the subcommittee's recommendations.

Most districts have inservice training for all staff at the beginning of each school year. Suggested topics for inservice training related to crisis intervention include:

- School climate: attention to low-level violence
  - Sexual harassment and bullying
- Lines of communication and reporting incidents
  - School policy, reviewing rules and consequences
- Improving communication skills
  - Listening skills inservice (see Chapter 3)
- Violence: How to deescalate a potential problem
  - See Overhead 3.2 in Chapter 3
  - See Handout 1.3 in Chapter 1
- Preventing burnout and handling stress (refer to Chapter 7)

INVENTORY OF STAFF SKILLS

All school employees have hidden skills related to crisis intervention that remain unrecognized and untapped. Every school should develop an inventory of staff skills (see Worksheet 6.1). Keeping an updated inventory of staff skills provides the principal and crisis team with a list of potential inhouse resources. Additional staff resources, particularly language skills, may be helpful in meeting the needs of students and families during a crisis. Considering employee skills when formulating crisis plans strengthens the school's resources and gives a greater level of confidence in meeting immediate needs. It is suggested that each school use Worksheet 6.1 merely as an example. Other questions may be added to provide a better fit with the unique needs of the school and community.

GUIDELINES FOR INVOLVING STAFF IN CRISIS INTERVENTION

The following list provides suggestions for involving all school adults in supporting crisis intervention:

1. Define school leadership/lines of authority. Each adult in the school must know who is responsible for what. This information should be available for easy reference. Highlight the specific responsibilities of each adult. Make sure each adult knows to whom he or she reports during an emergency.

2. Define duties. Review basic information and provide handouts for easy reference. To assist staff in providing support to students, review examples of what to say and what not to say. Use basic examples and role-play to practice the skill. Zero in on the most important information. Provide a one-page handout with key points.

3. Explain critical situations that would require a staff member to refer a student to an administrator or a professional. Using specific examples, practice these situations. Check for understanding by carefully reviewing these scenarios, in particular, (a) reporting suspected abuse, (b) requesting assistance for a potentially suicidal student, and (c) alerting supervisors or administrators about school safety concerns.

4. Define steps for reporting emergency information to a supervisor or administrator in charge. Designate to whom to report, when to report concerns, and how to report concerns. Provide a one-page handout listing these responsibilities.

5. Form teams of staff and teachers, making sure each group has an experienced leader. Periodically, review team assignments to ensure that team members work well together.

6. During staff meetings or inservice meetings, schedule brief practice sessions for "what if?" crisis scenarios. Training may include brief video vignettes followed by a group discussion. Handouts of designated responsibilities should be reviewed on a regular basis.

7. After a school crisis, schedule time for all adults to review and process what happened. This exchange provides an opportunity for members to bond as a group. Be sensitive to the emotional needs of those who assisted with the crisis. Acknowledge appreciation for staff support in participating in crisis intervention.

8. To encourage feedback and suggestions from staff and teachers, provide a suggestion box in the office or break room. Their suggestions will help improve the crisis plan.

SUGGESTED READING

Morgan, J., & Ashbaker, B. Y. (2001). *A teacher's guide to working with paraeducators and other classroom aides.* Alexandria, VA: Association for Supervision and Curriculum Development.

This 102-page book contains information about assisting paraprofessionals and teachers to cooperate, learn roles and duties, and improve relationships.

WEBSITE

www.nea.org/esphome/documents/drivers.pdf

This National Education Association website has a downloadable version of a bus driver booklet (17 pages).

Crisis Intervention

SKILLS INVENTORY

Name: _____

Job title: _____

Date: _____

Contact information: Phone # _____

Emergency # _____

E-mail address: _____

Do you speak another language? (Indicate language[s] and degree of fluency.)

Please list your experiences and training in first aid or medical training.

Please list your previous experiences with emergency situations.

If needed, would you be willing to assist with a classroom of students identified as having special needs?

In the event of a school crisis, what special abilities, services, or equipment could you offer?

List concerns you may have about assisting with a school crisis.

List your suggestions for improving crisis intervention in our school.

7

Avoiding Burnout

Taking Care of Yourself

MELISSA ALLEN HEATH *and* BART LYMAN

A PERSONAL EXAMPLE OF BURNOUT

A school psychologist who served on a district crisis team for 8 years shares this story:

"I thought back over my past month of experiences. As part of my job, I was on the school district crisis team. It had been a particularly difficult month: two suicides and a drive-by shooting. As a school psychologist, in addition to my regular responsibilities, I also had a particularly challenging load of counseling cases.

"I was tired. It had been weeks since I had felt rested. My dreams were filled with frustrating situations. I dreamed of driving and never getting to my destination, hunting for an important paper and never finding it, and entering a store shopping for bread, then forgetting what I needed to purchase. I was surprised that lately I woke up dreading the thought of going to work. I used to jump out of bed each day, excited to face new challenges.

"I remember driving down the road after getting ready for work one morning, thinking of my 'to do' list for the day. I knew I would never be able to get through the list. My stomach was aching. I reached for my antacid tablets. I never had time for breakfast anymore.

"I looked at my watch. My muscles tensed. I had to be to work in 15 minutes. I heaved a sigh. The car in front of me was going too slowly. I felt impatient.

"Then I saw a dead squirrel in the middle of the road. Everything stopped for me. I caught my breath and started to sob. It was completely out of character for me. I did not cry over things like this. What was wrong with me? Even though I knew this was just a squirrel, I could not stop sobbing. I had an overwhelming feeling of futility and despair.

"As strange as it may sound, until seeing that dead squirrel, I did not realize the emotional toll my job was taking on my well-being. In the past, when others needed emotional support, I was the strong one. Now I was the one needing support. After consulting with several crisis team members, I knew I was experiencing burnout. I immediately took steps to reduce my stress and bring my life back into balance."

WHAT IS BURNOUT?

The definition for *burnout*, as well as the symptoms associated with it, have evolved over the past three decades. Initially burnout was part of mental health terminology in the 1970s; it was used to describe the condition of patients who were emotionally and physically worn out from chronic stress and demands of daily life. In extreme cases, the individual lacked the energy to complete even the most basic tasks of everyday living.

Based on Freudenberger's (1974) research, new workers in alternative health care settings took their jobs very seriously. They were more apt to feel the personal effects of stress than were older, more experienced workers. Coming into a new job with high hopes and ideals, new workers soon discovered that their work was less appreciated and less fulfilling than originally anticipated. Summarizing Freudenberger's work in one sentence: Stress leading to burnout occurs when lofty idealism hits the harsh and brutal road of realism.

The psychiatric term burnout soon expanded to include those who were mentally and physically overwhelmed in the helping professions, particularly those involved in crisis intervention work. The stress associated with providing mental health care became a problem in 1960s and early 1970s as patient care was deinstitutionalized. The number of patients in state mental hospitals decreased drastically. The majority of individuals suffering with mental health problems was removed from state hospital care and turned over to outpatient services in local communities. This huge shift revolutionized mental health care in America. Crisis hotlines manned by volunteers became popular in attempts to assist with the overwhelming mental health needs.

Others suffering similar stress in meeting the extreme demands of emergency care included policemen, firemen, hospital emergency room workers, and emergency medical technician volunteers. These individuals, working daily with intense life-and-death situations, frequently exhibited symptoms of burnout. Researchers began to look at the effects of stress, noting the incredible toll stress takes on an individual who is overwhelmed with emotional and physical demands.

Burnout, however, is not limited in scope to one individual's isolated discomfort; employers, coworkers, and the public all feel the effects of burnout. Across all occupations, employers feel the monetary effects of employee burnout. Consequences of burnout include lower quality and quantity of work due to decreased commitment to responsibilities, high turnover, increased sick days, and low employee morale.

FACTORS THAT INCREASE STRESS

Every profession has some degree of stress. Deadlines for projects, daily demands, personal and professional responsibilities, conflicts with coworkers, and an increased emphasis on accountability all add to an individual's stress. Although a healthy amount of stress can lead to increased performance and sharpened skills, there is a point at which stress becomes detrimental to an individual's personal and professional life. At this point stress becomes counterproductive, taking a heavy toll on the individual's well-being.

Burnout in the helping and teaching professions has more to do with overwhelming emotional demands than heavy physical demands. Administrators, teachers, staff, and mental health professionals are prone to burnout partially because of their idealistic desire to make a difference in students' lives. Frequently several students in each classroom are in a state of crisis, their situations demanding immediate attention. Often their needs are complex and not easily or readily resolved. Over time the demands of the needy overwhelm the emotional resources of the helper. This scenario is all too typical.

It is important to remember that burnout occurs because of two factors: the nature of the job and the nature of the person. Some jobs are more stressful and some people are more vulnerable. What makes a stressful job? Job factors contributing to burnout may include rigid deadlines, long hours, ambiguous roles, mundane and repetitive tasks, unclear or conflicting expectations, heavy responsibilities, intense demands, limited control, unfair conditions, dangerous conditions, poor administrative leadership, inadequate support, limited recognition, or unpleasant social interactions.

Individuals most susceptible to burnout are those who have difficulty maintaining a healthy balance, finding a midpoint, avoiding the extreme. However, no one is invincible. Given the right set of circumstances, anyone could fall victim to experiencing symptoms of burnout. Personal characteristics predisposing a worker to burnout may include holding to high ideals of helping others and making a difference; expecting perfection of themselves and others; focusing on details rather than the big picture; needing and demanding order and control, rigid/inflexible; difficulty setting appropriate boundaries in relationships; overly desirous of pleasing others, overly sensitive to criticism; or ascribing to a strong work ethic involving excessive responsibility and industriousness. Although many of these characteristics are good in moderation, the problem arises when they are carried to an extreme, thereby creating imbalance.

Personal characteristics become more pronounced in certain work environments. Likewise, work environments are greatly influenced by an individual's personal characteristics. For instance, as previously stated, caring individuals seek out jobs in which they feel they can make a difference. Schools would certainly be a very different place if this were not the case. Rather than separating work environment and personal characteristics into two separate factors, it is more accurate to conceptualize burnout as occurring because of the relationship between characteristics of the job and characteristics of the individual.

SYMPTOMS OF BURNOUT

Symptoms of burnout typically have a slow onset, almost indiscernible to the affected individual. Smoldering in the background, burnout gradually expands, squeezing out an individual's enthusiasm for his or her job and for life, in general.

In order to avoid burnout, it is important to understand the symptoms—what burnout looks and feels like. First and foremost, symptoms of burnout occur on a continuum of severity, becoming visible when the individual's inner struggles erupt into pronounced and recognizable behavior. When an individual is experiencing burnout, he or she may act and feel differently. His or her responses to situations may surprise coworkers. For instance, a previously calm person may become irritable and lash out at a coworker. Table 7.1 lists several changes to consider when self-evaluating for burnout. To detect burnout, monitor symptoms in four areas: behavioral, physical, social, and emotional (James & Gilliland, 2001, p. 616).

KEEPING YOURSELF EMOTIONALLY HEALTHY

School crisis teams and those assisting with crisis intervention are susceptible to burnout not only because they are exposed to the traumatic event, but also because they "rub shoulders" with adults and students who are struggling to survive those events. Crisis team members may have a difficult time distancing themselves from the crisis. It is difficult for them to avoid personalizing the demands, stress, and pressures associated with the crisis.

Teachers and staff are also highly susceptible to burnout for the same reasons. On a daily basis they interact with, and assist, students who are experiencing trauma or difficulties. Burnout is almost unavoidable.

This seeming inevitability of burnout raises the question: What can crisis teams, teachers, and staff do to *avoid* burnout? The good news is there are ways to reduce stress

TABLE 7.1. Symptoms of Burnout

Watch for *changes* in these four areas:

Behavioral	Physical	Social	Emotional
Hyperactive or less active	Fatigue	Unpredictable	Overwhelmed
Complaining	Sleep problems	Impersonal/detached	Indifferent
Hypersensitive to stimuli; jumpy	Nightmares	Avoidant	Insensitive
	Muscle tension	Withdrawn	Numb
Extreme reactions: uncontrolled/overcontrolled	Stomachaches	Lacking personal limits	Irritable, edgy
	Headaches	Intolerant	Moody
Forgetful, preoccupied	Chronic illness	Distrustful	Cynical
Compulsive	Weight loss or gain	Controlling	Depressed
	Difficulty concentrating		Anxious
			Hopeless/helpless
			Guilty, inadequate

and protect or "inoculate" oneself against the harmful effects of burnout (see Handout 7.1 at the end of the chapter).

Evaluate Your Strengths and Weaknesses

Know Your Limitations

Awareness of personal vulnerabilities allows us to evaluate which aspects of crisis intervention might overwhelm our coping resources and helps us manage our level of participation in the crisis, thus (one hopes) avoiding burnout. For example, some individuals have the ability to remain calm and collected during a crisis, virtually unaffected by disorder and commotion. Others are highly agitated by noise and confusion. Because there are many ways to assist during a crisis, individuals should consider where their strengths can be best utilized. Likewise, they should be aware of circumstances that could overwhelm them.

Know Your Triggers for Stress

Personal experiences also affect our ability to cope with stress during a crisis situation. We all have painful memories that may be triggered during a crisis. Personal memories of accidents, deaths, or other tragedies increase our vulnerability to stress and burnout. For instance, those who have lost a family member to suicide may have particularly strong emotions triggered by a student or teacher's suicide. When details of a crisis mirror personal experiences, those assisting with the crisis may be overwhelmed with their own emotional reaction. Wanting to assist but not emotionally ready to face a situation, they may overreact, reducing their ability to help others. Avoid this undesirable scenario by knowing your triggers for stress.

Listen to Your Body

To monitor levels of stress, it is important to listen to your body. Physical health greatly affects mental health. If you are tired and irritable from lack of sleep, you will be at a greater risk for burnout. It is also important to eat a well-balanced diet and to maintain healthy habits. Although these suggestions may sound fundamental, they are very important in preventing burnout.

Share and Delegate Responsibilities

Another suggestion for preventing burnout is to monitor your level of responsibility. Nothing wears an individual down faster than feeling like he or she is carrying the weight of the world. Joining together as a team of coworkers is not only a good suggestion, it is essential. Sharing responsibilities and appreciating each person's contribution to the team strengthens the school's crisis plan. Schools are safer and students are more supported when every adult participates in carrying the load of responsibilities. In making and refining crisis plans, it is important to spread out responsibilities so each adult contributes and is accountable for his or her contribution.

Maintain Appropriate Boundaries

One of the best words in the English language is "no." However, teachers, staff, and mental health professionals typically have a difficult time saying this word. We often lose ourselves in our commitments to too many causes. This overcommitment adds fuel to burnout.

Becoming overinvolved in student problems is another common mistake for those who work with students and families. It is helpful to think of this scenario. Imagine yourself standing at the edge of a deep hole. A person in the hole is reaching up to you, asking for your help. The person desperately wants you to pull him or her out the deep hole. However, here is the danger: If you get too close, the person will pull you down inside the hole. You cannot pull out the person if you get too close to the edge. You have to stay back and ask for others to come and help you. When you become too involved personally, you fall into the hole with the victim. This is not to suggest that you remain unfeeling and keep too much distance from the problem. However, you must find a healthy balance. You do not own another person's problems. You can provide support, but you cannot fix another person's problems. If you get too involved, you will burn out quickly. It is important to have confidence in each individual's capacity to heal, learn, and grow from his or her experiences.

Another suggestion to prevent burnout is to guard family time and weekends as periods of relaxation. Try to leave student problems and other school issues at school. When leaving the school building, take a deep breath and switch your mind into another mode, free time. When you return on Monday, school problems left behind on Friday will be patiently waiting inside the school. By separating your home life and your school life, you will greatly reduce the risk of burnout.

Develop Support Networks

Establishing support networks and participating in a variety of activities are vital in reducing stress. It is important to feel connected with others. Work-related support could include participating in peer mentoring programs and increasing your opportunities for collaboration by attending professional associations and professional development activities. More informally, individuals can reduce stress by socializing with family and friends and attending social activities outside of work. Strengthening spiritual connections provides another source of social support.

On a group level, debriefings provide an opportunity for crisis team members to bond and support one another. After a school crisis, the crisis response team should hold an "operational debriefing." This is an excellent way to pull together and address everyone's emotional needs after a crisis. Team debriefing assists in building group cohesiveness and addressing stress levels of group members (Everly & Mitchell, 2000). Adapted from Everly and Mitchell's model, Johnson (2000) suggests the following format for team debriefing in schools: introductory phase, fact phase, assessment phase, and interpretation phase.

The introductory phase sets the stage for the group meeting by outlining the parameters of the meeting and who is in charge. In the school setting it is important to use the existing structure of leadership, utilizing the principal as the person in charge.

The fact phase provides an opportunity to discuss what actually happened. Additionally, it gives members an opportunity to explore what they observed from their perspective and to find a semblance of order to the events.

The assessment phase encourages members to discuss how individuals tackled specific problems that arose during the crisis, which strategies worked, and which strategies did not work.

The last phase, interpretation, gives team members the chance to "pull it all together" and place the situation in perspective. With the information provided by group members, the team has the opportunity to plan for the future and make improvements on existing strategies.

The primary focus of the group debriefing should be on supporting members and building connections. Increasing emotional support among crisis team members prevents burnout.

Stress-Reducing Activities

Most doctors would endorse this statement: Stress greatly contributes to the onset of illness and disease. Stress is one of the most common reasons for leaving jobs. In fact, when offered a "menu" of topics for possible inservice training, staff and teachers overwhelmingly choose "stress reduction" as the number-one topic of choice. Teachers and staff readily acknowledge the need to reduce stress. Based on their feedback, stress caused them the greatest dissatisfaction at work.

One way to reduce stress is by increasing physical activity and exercising regularly. In fact, physical exercise continues to be one of the most effective research-based interventions for stress reduction. Mental health workers and medical professionals agree that mild and moderate exercise assists the body in overcoming stress, anxiety, and depression. Exercising benefits both mental and physical well-being. The trick is to find the type of physical activity that fits your schedule, budget, and lifestyle. Exercising with a friend increases the likelihood of carrying out an exercise plan.

If someone asks what your hobbies are and you pause to think before responding, you need to expand your horizons and develop a passion for a hobby. Think about what you previously enjoyed doing in your spare time. Hobbies come in many forms: knitting, reading, drawing, photography, and so on. Some people become an expert on a topic, such as World War II. Whatever form it takes, a hobby can provide pleasure and satisfaction, which buffer the effects of stress.

Planning a vacation and taking time away from work and responsibilities is another way to reduce stress. Even when the vacation is in the distant future, the hope and dream alone are enough to help reduce stress. Get books from the library. Go to a travel agency. Look on the Internet for travel deals.

Finally, remember to laugh, a wonderful way to reduce stress. Take time to go to a comedy, either a play or a movie. Watch a TV show that makes you laugh. Keep a "humor" file in your desk. Cut out jokes and cartoons to share with others. Look for humor all around you. Schools provide a veritable smorgasbord of humor. Feast on the delicious situations as they arise. Check out some good children's books from the library. The possibilities are endless.

Staff and Teacher Training Activity

Review the following example:

Teresa is a fourth-grade teaching assistant. She has been an employee of the district for the past 5 years. Last year her school district honored her with the Support Staff of the Year award. She is soft-spoken and patient with students in the classroom.

Teresa is a single parent raising four young children. She is actively involved in the local Hispanic community. She frequently stays after school to tutor children who are behind in reading, particularly those who speak Spanish. She is frequently called upon to assist with Spanish translation for parent–teacher conferences. She has a reputation of looking after kids who are having difficulties with school and with their families.

She goes out of her way to help others. Last year, when neighbors lost their home in a fire, she took the family into her own home for several weeks until other arrangements were made. Although she is not a member of the crisis team, she has assisted with deescalating fights and has a reputation for being a good listener. Students frequently go to Teresa with personal problems.

Until this year, Teresa was always on time for work; she was very dependable. This year, however, Teresa seems different. Her supervising teacher, Mr. Adams, reports having a poor working relationship with Teresa. According to him, she spends too much time talking with students about nonacademic topics. For instance, he recently complained that Teresa was spending far too much time with one student who reportedly has a history of abuse. Mr. Adams complains that she is not assisting students with academic work. Another complaint is that Teresa speaks too much Spanish with students. He believes the students should be speaking more English in the classroom.

Teresa is arriving late to work and has called in sick several days this month. She is not reviewing students' homework or completing the classroom paperwork. Mr. Adams made an appointment with the principal to discuss Teresa's situation.

After reviewing this example, discuss the following questions with teachers and staff.

- Identify stressors in Teresa's personal life.
- Identify job stressors.
- Identify recent changes in Teresa's behavior.
- Putting yourself in Teresa's place, what would you do to prevent this situation from worsening?
- Taking ideas from Handout 7.1, "Preventing Burnout," list some things Teresa could do to improve her situation.

CONCLUSION

In assisting with crisis intervention, make sure you feel that you are a part of a team, whether a district crisis team or part of the school staff. There are always others who can share the burden of helping students through difficult times. After assisting with a crisis situation, take time to speak with other professionals or friends who are emotionally supportive and caring.

No one is immune to burnout. It is important to recognize symptoms and increase self-awareness of the personal and job-related stressors that contribute to burnout. Likewise, it is equally important to maintain balance in your life, ensuring that there are enough positives to outweigh the negatives. Take time to relax and enjoy stress-reducing activities, particularly physical exercise.

SUGGESTED READING

Huebner, E. S., Gilligan, T. D., & Cobb, H. (2002). Best practices in preventing and managing stress and burnout. In A. Thomas & J. Grimes (Eds.), *Best practices in school psychology* (Vol. 4, pp. 173–182). Bethesda, MD: National Association of School Psychologists.

James, R. K., & Gilliland, B. E. (2001). Human services workers in crisis: Burnout. In *Crisis intervention strategies* (4th ed., pp. 609–646). Belmont, CA: Brooks/Cole.

Johnson, K. (2000). Taking care of yourself. In *School crisis management: A hands-on guide to training crisis response teams* (pp. 87–92). Alameda, CA: Hunter House.

Maslach, C., & Goldberg, J. (1998). Prevention of burnout: New perspectives. *Applied and Preventative Psychology, 7,* 63–74.

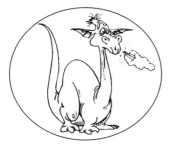

Preventing Burnout: Keeping Yourself Emotionally Healthy

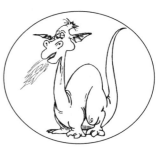

- **Realistically evaluate your strengths and weaknesses.**
  - Know your limitations.
  - Know your triggers for stress.
  - Listen to your body.

- **Share and delegate responsibilities to coworkers.**
  - Know that you are part of a team.
  - Appreciate the contributions of others.

- **Maintain appropriate boundaries.**
  - Say "no."
  - Distance yourself from student issues.
  - Guard your family time and weekends.

- **Develop support networks..**
  - Socialize with family and friends.
  - Strengthen your spiritual connections.
  - Consult with other professionals.

- **Take time for stress-reducing activities.**
  - Exercise
  - Hobbies
  - Vacations
  - Laughter

Appendix A

Free Crisis Intervention Resources from the Substance Abuse and Mental Health Services Administration

The following table provides information about materials available free of charge through the U.S. Department of Health and Human Services. For more information, go to *www.samhsa.gov*.

SAMSHA material	Publication date	Summary	Would we recommend this for your school?
Communicating in a Crisis: Risk Communication Guidelines for Public Officials	2002	Provides instruction on how to communicate during a disaster or crisis.	Useful for the person in charge of dealing with the media during a crisis at school.
Developing Cultural Competence in Disaster Mental Health Programs	2003	Discusses cultural competence as it relates to crisis response. Gives nine principles to follow when developing a culturally sensitive plan for crisis intervention.	The first section would be very useful in a school setting. The second section (nine principles) is also helpful, but parts need to be adjusted to apply to schools.
Disaster Mental Health: Crisis Counseling Programs for the Rural Community	1999	Gives information about organizing a crisis response program in rural communities. Details phases of dealing with disaster and special considerations for rural communities.	More of a community guide, but some good information if your school is located in a rural community.
Evaluation of the Comprehensive Community Mental Health Services for Children and Their Families Program: Annual Report to Congress: 1999	1999	Presents statistics and information about the success of federally funded community mental health services for children. Provides descriptions of participating community program models.	Helpful if searching for a model to follow.
Fact Sheets		SAMHSA has several fact sheets dealing with specific issues related to the mental health of all populations.	Valuable resources.
Field Manual for Mental Health and Human Service Workers in Major Disasters	2000 (reprinted in 2002)	Summary of *Training Manual for Mental Health and Human Service Workers in Major Disasters*. Includes questions to ask as well as do's and don'ts of helping others during disaster.	Yes, a useful reference for any school personnel.

(continued)

SAMSHA material	Publication date	Summary	Would we recommend this for your school?
Mental Health: Culture, Race, and Ethnicity. A Supplement to Mental Health: A Report of the Surgeon General	2001	Present findings that, although prevalence of mental illness is not greater among minorities, availability and quality of mental health care are not as adequate. Because of this inadequacy, minorities with mental illness may experience greater disability. Specifically, discusses four minority groups. Includes suggestions or goals for improving mental health care for minorities.	Yes.
National Strategies for Suicide Prevention: Goals and Objectives for Action	2001	Starts with a history of the government's role in suicide prevention efforts. Lists common aspects of effective suicide prevention programs. Discusses national suicide prevention goals, then gives suggestions for how to evaluate local prevention efforts. Describes specific research programs in progress. Provides a list of additional resources.	Yes, but there is *a lot* of information.
Psychosocial Issues for Children and Families in Disasters: A Guide for the Primary Care Physician	1995	Written primarily for physicians, this guide details how children may react in times of crisis. Briefly describes stages of a disaster as well as common reactions during each stage. Gives physicians suggestions for how to help.	Yes. Though it is written for physicians, the descriptions and tips would be useful for any helping professional.
Recovering Your Mental Health: Dealing with the Effects of Trauma	2002	Gives a brief definition of trauma with a list of possible reactions. Includes several helpful tips for healing from traumatic events. Also includes a list of other resources.	Yes. This could be given to teachers. It could also be used as a self-help resource in high school counseling centers.
Suicide Fast Facts	2002	Quarter sheet of paper with a few facts about suicide as well as a list of resources.	Yes.
Systems of Care: Promising Practices in Children's Mental Health: Learning From Families: Identifying Service Strategies for Success	2001	Presents findings from a quantitative study about which service delivery characteristics were most helpful in facilitating desired changes among families with children who had behavioral or emotional disorders.	Yes, useful for school mental health professionals.
Systems of Care: Promising Practices in Children's Mental Health: The Role of Education in a System of Care: Effectively Serving Children with Emotional or Behavioral Disorders	2001	Discusses the need for school involvement when treating children with emotional or behavioral disorders. Presents effective program models and delineates underlying principles of those models. Provides suggestions for implementing school-based systems of care and addresses how to overcome barriers to the implementation of programs.	Yes.

(continued)

SAMSHA material	Publication date	Summary	Would we recommend this for your school?
Training Manual for Mental Health and Human Service Workers in Major Disasters	2000	Includes sections on responses to disaster, reactions of specific groups (e.g., ethnic, children), and stress response and management. Also offers suggestions for training. A course outline and training overheads are provided.	Yes, useful for a school's crisis response team.
What You Need to Know about Youth Violence Prevention	2002	Discusses research and trends of youth violence. Lists common risk factors as well as successful prevention programs.	Yes.
Youth Violence: A Report of the Surgeon General: Executive Summary	2001	Summarizes the Surgeon General's report on youth violence. Includes a list of myths about youth violence. Also briefly describes findings about trends in youth violence, pathways to youth violence, risk and protective factors, preventing youth violence, and a vision for the future.	Yes.

Appendix B

Additional Books for Bibliotherapy

<u>Tolerance for diversity</u>

The Other Side by Jacqueline Woodson
ISBN 0-39923-116-1

A young black girl, Clover, has been told never to cross the fence separating her yard from the neighbor's (who are white). The daughter of the family across the fence is always sitting on it. Clover finally gets the courage to talk to her, and they become friends.

Yoko by Rosemary Wells
ISBN 0-78680-395-9

Yoko's mother makes sushi for lunch. Other students make fun of her. Later, the teacher plans an international day when each student brings a dish from a different country.

The Storm by Marc Harshman
ISBN 0-52565-150-0

Jonathan felt different because he was in a wheelchair. When a tornado comes to town and he is alone, he finds the strength to overcome his fear.

<u>Parents with mental illness</u>

Mama One, Mama Two by Patricia Maclachlan
ASIN 0898456614

A little girl is living with "mama two" because "mama one" is depressed. Describes the child's experience in foster care, ending with the hope that "mama one" will be able to take care of her again soon.

<u>Chronic illness</u>

Child of the Morning by Barbara Corcoran
ASIN 0689308760

Susan spends her summer working with a theater group. She struggles with "odd spells" that are not explained until a new doctor moves to town.

Singing with Momma Lou by Linda Jacobs Altman
ISBN 1-58430-040-X

Tamika visits her grandmother, who has Alzheimer's, every week. She feels frustrated that Momma Lou doesn't remember her. Tamika decides that she will try to help her remember.

<u>Friendship problems</u>

Just as Long as We're Together by Judy Blume
ISBN 0-44021-094-1

Two friends become three when a new girl moves into the neighborhood. They face school and personal struggles together.

Simon and Molly Plus Hester by Lisa Jahn-Clough
ISBN 0-61808-220-4

Simon and Molly are best friends until Hester moves into their neighborhood. Molly starts to play with Hester, and Simon feels left out. He eventually learns that all three can be friends.

<u>Financial difficulties</u>

A Chair for My Mother by Vera Williams
ISBN 0-68804-074-8

After their home is destroyed by fire, Rosa's family saves every spare penny to buy a comfortable chair where Rosa's mother can sit at the end of long days at work.

If the Shoe Fits by Gary Soto
ISBN 0-39923-420-9

Rigo hates hand-me-downs and is particularly excited when he gets new shoes for his birthday. When the shoes no longer fit, Rigo finds new appreciation for hand-me-downs as he gives his shoes to his uncle.

(continued)

Overcoming fear

Mirette on the High Wire
by Emily Arnold McCully
ISBN 0-69811-443-4

Mirette meets the Great Bellini, a master wire-walker. Little does she know how she will help him overcome great fear to perform once again.

The Princesses of Bamarre
by Gail Carlson Levine
ISBN 0-06440-966-X

Addie is the scared princess who is protected by her sister Meryl. But it is Meryl who gets sick and Addie who must face her fears to find a way to help.

Bullying

Stop Picking on Me, a 1st Look at Bullying
by Pat Thomas
ISBN 0-76411-461-1

This book helps children understand what bullying is and what it might look like. It also helps the reader to understand some reasons why a child might bully others. It ends by giving children practical and healthy solutions to being bullied.

The Kweeks of Kookatumdee by Bill Peet
ISBN 0-39548-656-4

Without enough "ploppolop" fruit trees to feed them and facing Jed the overgrown bully, the "kweeks" fear they will starve until Quentin makes a great discovery.

King of the Cooties by Debbie Dadey
ISBN 0-80277-622-1

Nate is excited when a new boy, Donald, moves into the neighborhood until the class bully begins to call Donald "King of the Cooties." Nate and Donald have to figure out how to stop the bully from bothering them.

Anger

When Sophie Gets Angry, Really, Really Angry by Molly Bang
ISBN 0-59018-979-4

When Sophie gets angry, she yells, runs, and cries. Many things help her calm down.

How Are You Peeling? by Saxton Freymann and Joost Ellfers
ISBN 0-43910-431-9

Cleverly sculptured to resemble facial expressions, vegetables and fruits depict a wide range of feelings and emotions.

Mean Soup by Betsy Everitt
ISBN 0-15200-227-8

When Horace has a terrible day, his mother helps him express himself while cooking dinner.

Abuse

It's MY Body by Lori Freeman
ISBN 0-94399-003-3

This book helps young children begin to understand personal boundaries, defining the difference between good touch and bad touch.

One of the Problems of Everett Anderson by Lucille Clifton and Ann Grifalconi
ISBN 0-80505-201-1

Everett is worried about his new friend, who comes to school with bruises and cuts. His friend tells him he can't tell anyone. Everett finally tells his mom, who reports it and comforts Everett.

Divorce

She's Not My Real Mother by Judith Vigna
ISBN 0-80757-340-X

A little boy doesn't like his dad's new wife until a day at the zoo, when he gets lost and she finds him.

Dear Mr. Henshaw by Beverly Clearly
ISBN 0-38070-958-9

Leigh writes several letters to an author, Mr. Henshaw. The book explores his feelings about his parents' divorce.

(continued)

Two Homes by Claire Masurel
ISBN 0-76361-984-1

Explores the adjustment of having two homes after a divorce.

Mama and Daddy Bear's Divorce
by Cornelia Maude Spelman
ISBN 0-80755-222-4

Dina Bear is scared when her parents divorce.

Death and grief

Nana Upstairs, Nana Downstairs
by Tomie dePaola
ISBN 0-39923-108-0

Tommy spends time with both his grandmother and his great-grandmother until the day "Nana Upstairs" dies. Based on a true story.

Geranium Morning by E. Sandy Powell
ISBN 0-87614-542-X

Two friends who both lose their parents find commonalities as they cycle through the grieving process.

After Charlotte's Mom Died
by Cornelia Spelman
ISBN 0-80750-196-4

When Charlotte's mom dies, she feels scared, sad, and mad. She and her father visit a therapist, who helps them understand feelings related to loss.

Someone Special Died by Joan Prestine
ISBN 0-86653-929-8

This book explores a young girl's feelings when someone she loved has died and shows how she learns to remember the person who died.

Bridge to Terabithia by Katherine Patterson
ISBN 0-06440-184-7

Jess dreams of being the fastest runner in fifth grade until a new girl moves into the neighborhood. Leslie is a tomboy and is faster than Jess. Despite this, they become friends and create an imaginary world in the woods. One day, tragedy strikes and Leslie dies. Jess faces the loss and learns to cope.

Missing May by Cynthia Rylant
ISBN 0-53105-996-0

Summer lives with her Aunt May and Uncle Ob. When Aunt May dies, Cletus comes and helps Summer and Uncle Ob learn to deal with May's death.

Parent problems

When They Fight by Kathryn White
ISBN 1-89081-746-5

A young badger speaks metaphorically about how he feels when his parents fight. The story points out that even when his parents fight, they still love their little badger.

Suicide

Artie's Brief: The Whole Truth and Nothing But by Christi Killien
ASIN 0380711087

Artie's friend at school is being picked on. His friend reminds him of an older brother who committed suicide. As he tries to help his friend, he learns to understand his feelings related to the suicide.

Up on Cloud Nine by Anne Fine
ISBN 0-38573-009-8

Ian's best friend, Stolly, is in a coma at the hospital. He appears to have fallen (or jumped) out a window. Ian tries to figure out what happened.

But I Didn't Say Good-Bye: For Parents and Professionals Helping Child Suicide Survivors by Barbara Rubel
ISBN 1-89290-600-7

This book helps professionals and others working with children survivors of suicide. Includes additional sources of information.

Someone I Loved Died by Suicide: A Story for Child Survivors and Those Who Care for Them by Doreen Cammarata
ISBN 0-97093-329-0

The story in the book is written to help children suffering through loss understand the grieving process as well as other emotions related to suicide.

References

Allen, M., Sheen, D., Jones, N., Heaton, E., Young, E., & Gstettenbauer, A. (2003). *Bibliotherapy: A resource to facilitate emotional healing and growth*. Manuscript submitted for publication.

Allen, M., Stott, K. A., Jones, N., Heaton, E., & Gstettenbauer, A. (2003, April). *Bibliotherapy: A resource for strengthening children's coping skills after a crisis*. Mini-Skills Workshop Presented at the 35th National Association of School Psychologists Annual Convention, Toronto, Canada.

Amato, P. R. (2001). Children of divorce in the 1990s: An update of the Amato and Keith (1991) meta-analysis. *Journal of Family Psychology, 15*(3), 355–370.

American Association of University Women. (2001). *Hostile hallways: Bullying, teasing, and sexual harassment in school*. Washington, DC: Author. (Available from *www.aauw.org*)

Armstrong, M. (1991). Cross-cultural issues in responding to a tragedy: The Stockton schoolyard shootings. In J. Sandoval (Ed.), *Resources in crisis intervention: School, family, and community applications* (pp. 97–99). Silver Spring, MD: National Association of School Psychologists.

Berk, L. E. (2003). *Child development* (6th ed). Boston: Allyn & Bacon.

Bracken, B. A., & McCallum, R. S. (1998). *Universal nonverbal intelligence test*. Itasca, IL: Riverside.

Brandon, R. (2003). Family matters: Mental health of children and parents. Policy brief. University of Washington, Seattle. Human Services Policy Center. (ED478231)

Brock, S. E., & Sandoval, J. (1997). Suicidal ideation and behaviors. In G. G. Bear, K. M. Minke, & A. Thomas (Eds.), *Children's needs II: Development, problems and alternatives* (pp. 361–374). Bethesda, MD: National Association of School Psychologists.

Brock, S. E., Sandoval, J., & Lewis, S. (2001). *Preparing for crisis in the schools: A manual for building school crisis response teams* (2nd ed.). New York: Wiley.

Burns, B. J., & Hoagwood, K. (2002). *Community-based treatment for youth: Evidence-based interventions for severe emotional and behavioral disorders*. New York: Oxford University Press.

Canter, A. S., & Carroll, S. A. (Eds.). (1999). *Crisis prevention and response: A collection of NASP resources*. Bethesda, MD: National Association of School Psychologists.

Caplan, G. (1964). *Principles of preventive psychiatry*. New York: Basic Books.

Carroll, S. A. (1999). Emotional first-aid: A school's guide to crisis intervention. In A. S. Canter & S. A. Carroll (Eds.), *Crisis prevention and response: A collection of NASP resources* (pp. 109–110). Bethesda, MD: National Association of School Psychologists.

Coie, J. D., & Dodge, K. A. (1998). Aggression and antisocial behavior. In N. Eisenberg (Ed.), *Handbook of child psychology: Vol. 3, Social emotional and personality development* (5th ed., pp. 779–862). New York: Wiley.

Curtis, M. J., Grier, J. E. C., Abshier, D. W., Sutton, N. T., & Hunley, S. (2002). School psychology: Turning the corner into the twenty-first century. *Communique, 30* (8), 1, 5–6.

Curtis, M. J., Hunley, S. A., Walker, K. J., & Baker, A. C. (1999). Demographic characteristics and professional practices in school psychology. *School Psychology Review, 28,* 104–116.

Dacey, J. S., & Fiore, L. B. (2002). *Your anxious child: How parents and teachers can help anxiety in children*. New York: Wiley.

Doll, B., & Doll, C. (1997). *Bibliotherapy with young people: Librarians and mental health professionals working together*. Englewood, CO: Libraries Unlimited.

Doll, B., Zucker, S., & Brehm, K. (2004). *Resilient classrooms: Creating healthy environments for learning*. New York: Guilford Press.

Education Week. (2002). The relative risks of school travel: A national perspective and guidance for local community assessment. *Education Week, 21*(43). Retrieved August 7, 2002, from *www.nap.edu*

Elliot, S., Kratochwill, T., & Roach, A. (2003). Commentary: Implementing social–emotional and academic innovations: Reflections, reactions, and research. *School Psychology Review, 32*(3), 320–327.

Evans, G. W. (2004). The environment of childhood poverty. *American Psychologist, 59*(2), 77–92.

Everly, G. S., Jr., & Mitchell, J. T. (Eds.). (2000). *Critical incident stress management: Advanced group crisis interventions: A workbook*. Ellicott City, MD: International Critical Incident Stress Foundation.

Fitzgerald, H. (1992). *The grieving child: A parent's guide*. New York: Simon & Schuster.

Ford, D. Y. (2000). Multicultural literature and gifted black students: Promoting self-understanding, awareness, and pride. *Roeper Review, 22*(4), 235–240.

Forgan, J. (2002). Using bibliotherapy to teach problem-solving. *Intervention in School and Clinic, 38*(2), 75–82.

Freudenberger, H. J. (1974). Staff burn-out. *Journal of Social Issues, 30,* 159–165.

Frydenberg, E., & Lewis, R. (1999). The adolescent coping scale: Construct validity and what the instrument tells us. *Australian Journal of Guidance Counseling, 9,* 19–36.

Frydenberg, E., & Lewis, R. (2002). Adolescent well-being: Building young people's resources. In E. Frydenberg (Ed.), *Beyond coping: Meetings goals, vision and challenges* (pp. 175–194). Oxford, UK: Oxford University Press.

Guin, K. (2004, August 16). Chronic teacher turnover in urban elementary schools. *Education Policy Analysis Archives, 12*(42). Retrieved August 26, 2004, from *epaa.asu.edu/epaa/v12n42/v12n42.pdf*

Hetherington, E. M., & Stanley-Hagan, M. (1999). The adjustment of children with divorced parents: A risk and resiliency perspective. *Journal of Child Psychology and Psychiatry, 40*(1), 129–140.

Holmes, M. (2000). *A terrible thing happened*. Washington, DC: Magination Press.

James, R. K., & Gilliland, B. E. (2001). *Crisis intervention strategies* (4th ed.). Pacific Grove, CA: Brooks/Cole.

Johnson, K. (1998). *Trauma in the lives of children*. Alameda, CA: Hunter House.

Johnson, K. (2000). *School crisis management: A hands-on guide to training crisis response teams* (2nd ed.). Alameda, CA: Hunter House.

Kübler-Ross, E. (1969). *On death and dying.* New York: Macmillan.

Kupersmidt, J. B., & Dodge, K. A. (2004). *Children's peer relations: From development to intervention.* Washington, DC: American Psychological Association.

Lightfoot, J., Wright, S., & Sloper, P. (1999). Supporting pupils in mainstream school with an illness or disability: Young people's views. *Child: Care, Health and Development, 25*(4), 267–283.

Lindemann, E. (1944). Symptomatology and management of acute grief. *American Journal of Psychiatry, 101*, 141–148.

Lindemann, E. (1979). *Beyond grief: Studies in crisis intervention.* New York: Aronson.

Maleki, C., & Elliot, S. (2002). Children's social behaviors as predictors of academic achievement: A longitudinal analysis. *School Psychology Quarterly, 17*, 1–23.

Maslow, A. (1970). *Motivation and personality* (2nd ed). New York: Harper & Row.

Masten, A. S. (2001). Ordinary magic: Resilience processes in development. *American Psychologist, 56*, 227–238

McCarty, H., & Chalmers, L. (1997). Bibliotherapy intervention and prevention. *Teaching Exceptional Children, 29*, 12–17.

McIntyre, T. (1999). *Bibliotherapy.* Retrieved July 6, 2003, from *maxweber.hunter.cuny.edu/eres/ EDSPC715_MCINTYRE/Biblio.html*

National Center for Educational Statistics. (2002). *Public school student, staff, and graduate counts by state: School year 2000–2001.* Retrieved January 4, 2003, from *nces.ed.gov/pubs2002/ snf_report/*

National Institute of Child Health and Human Development. (2003). *America's children: Key national indicators of well-being, 2003.* Retrieved April 19, 2004, from *www.nichd.nih.gov/publications/pubs/childstats/americas03.htm*

National School Transportation Association. (2002a). *The ABC's of school busing.* Retrieved December 13, 2002, from *www.schooltrans.com/abc.htm*

National School Transportation Association. (2002b). *Did you know?* Retrieved December 13, 2002, from *www.schooltrans.com/didyouknow.htm*

Nickerson, E. (1975). Bibliotherapy: A therapeutic medium for helping children. *Psychotherapy: Theory, Research and Practice, 12*(3), 258–261.

Olweus, D. (1993). *Bullying at school: What we know and what we can do.* Malden, MA: Blackwell.

Pardeck, J. T. (1991). Using books to prevent and treat adolescent chemical dependency. *Adolescence, 26*, 201–208.

Pardeck, J. T. (1995). Bibliotherapy: An innovative approach for helping children. *Early Child Development and Care, 110*, 83–88.

Pardeck, J. T., & Pardeck, J. A. (1997) Recommended books for helping young children deal with social and developmental problems. *Early Child Development and Care, 136*, 57–63.

Pasko, J. R. (1994). Chicago—don't miss it. *Communique, 23*(4), 2.

Pedersen, P. B. (2003). Culturally biased assumptions in counseling psychology. *The Counseling Psychologist, 31*, 396–403.

Percy, M., (2003). Feeling loved, having friends to count on, and taking care of yourself: Minority children living in poverty describe what is "special" to them. *Journal of Children and Poverty, 9*(1), 55–70.

Poland, S., Pitcher, G., & Lazarus, P. J. (1999). Best practices in crisis intervention. In A. S. Canter & S. A. Carroll (Eds.), *Crisis prevention and response: A collection of NASP resources* (pp. 69–86). Bethesda, MD: National Association of School Psychologists.

Putallaz, M., & Bierman, K. L. (Eds.). (2004). *Aggression, antisocial behavior, and violence among girls: A developmental perspective.* New York: Guilford Press.

Richardson, C. D., & Rosen, L. A. (1999). School-based interventions for children of divorce. *Professional School Counseling, 3,* 21–26.

Romualdi, V., & Sandoval, J. (1995). Comprehensive school-linked services: Implications for school psychologists. *Psychology in the Schools, 12,* 306–317.

Ross, S. M., & Lowther, D. L. (2003). Impacts of the connect school reform design on classroom instruction, school climate, and student achievement in inner-city schools. *Journal of Education for Students Placed at Risk, 8*(2), 215–246.

Sandoval, J., & Brock, S. E. (1996). The school psychologists's role in suicide prevention. *School Psychology Quarterly, 11,* 169–185.

Steward, M. S. (2002). Illness: A crisis for children. In J. Sandoval (Ed.), *Handbook of crisis counseling, intervention, and prevention in the schools* (2nd ed., pp. 183–211). Mahwah, NJ: Erlbaum.

Striepling, S. H. (1997). The low-aggression classroom: A teacher's view. In A. P. Goldstein & J. C. Conoley (Eds.), *School violence intervention: A practical handbook* (pp. 23–45). New York: Guilford Press.

Sue, D. W., & Sue, D. (2003). *Counseling the culturally different: Theory and practice* (4th ed.). New York: Wiley.

Tu, W. (1999). *Using literature to help children cope with problems* (Report No. EDO-CS-99–09). Bloomington, IN: ERIC Clearinghouse on Reading, English and Communication. (ERIC Document Reproduction Service No. ED436008)

U.S. Bureau of the Census. (2001). *Statistical abstract of the United States.* Retrieved January 4, 2003, from *www.census.gov/prod/2002pubs/01statab/educ.pdf*

U.S. Bureau of the Census. (2002). *Statistical abstract of the United States: 2002.* Retrieved November 18, 2003, from *www.census.gov/prod/2003pubs/02statab/educ.pdf*

U.S. Department of Health and Human Services. (2000). *Healthy people 2010: Conference edition* (Vols. I and II). Washington, DC: Author.

U.S. Department of Health and Human Services. (2001). *National strategy for suicide prevention: Goals and objectives for action.* Rockville, MD: Author.

Velting, O., Setzer, N., & Albano, A. (2004). Update on and advances in assessment and cognitive-behavioral treatment of anxiety disorders in children and adolescents. *Professional Psychology, Research and Practice, 35*(1), 42–54.

Weinberg, R. B. (1989). Consultation and training with school-based crisis teams. *Professional Psychology: Research and Practice, 20,* 305–308.

Index

Abuse, 55, 81–82, 116, 117, 122, 123, 124
Acceptance, 83–84
Action plans, 48
Activities, classroom
  bibliotherapy; *see* Bibliotherapy
  communication, 99–100
  fear, 87–88
  feelings, 85–87, 91–92, 93–97
  getting to know you, 97–98
  group rules, defining, 90–91
  problem-solving, 100–101
  self-image, 101–102
  sexual harassment, 10
  student response to stress and trauma, 85–102
  teamwork, 98–99
  tolerance, 88–89
ADHD, 132
Adults, responsibilities of, 7, 28–29
Aggression. *See* Bullying
Anger, 83–84, 131–132, 141
Anxiety, 78, 130, 131, 132
Attention-Deficit/Hyperactivity Disorder (ADHD), 132

B

Behavior, stress/trauma and, 11–12
Bibliotherapy
  ADHD, 132
  anger, 141
  anxiety, 131, 132
  books, additional, 164–166
  bullying, 22, 135
  communication with parents, 68
  conflict resolution, 135, 140
  death, 134, 135
  Define "Normal" (Peters), 136
  definition, 65–66
  diversity, 66–67, 135, 136
  divorce, 134
  fear, 131
  financial difficulties, 137, 138, 139
  friendship, 133
  Gettin' through Thursday (Cooper), 137
  How to Lose All Your Friends (Carlson), 133
  Is It Right to Fight? (Thomas), 141
  Joey Pigza Swallowed the Key (Gantos), 132
  Lilly's Purple Plastic Purse (Henkes), 140
  literature selection, 66–67
  as a mental health tool, 64–65
  mental illness, 135, 136
  Money Hungry (Flake), 138
  My Louisiana Sky (Holt), 135
  Nobody Knew What to Do (McCain), 22
  obesity, 134
  parent problems, 134, 135
  physical symptoms of stress and, 68–69
  problem solving, 135
  professional referrals and, 68
  Ramona and Her Father (Cleary), 139
  stages of, 66
  stress/trauma, 68–69, 85
  teaching techniques, 67–68
  tolerance, 134, 135, 136
  When Addie Was Scared (Bailey), 131
  When Zachary Beaver Came to Town (Holt), 134
Body language, communication skills and, 47
Boundaries, burnout prevention and, 155
Bullying
  bibliotherapy, 135
  classroom activities, 9–10
  prevention of, 4–6
  resources, 13–22
  targeting of, 6–8
Burnout
  definition, 151
  effects of, 151–152
  prevention, 153–156
  resources, 158
  stress-reducing activities, 156
  symptoms, 153
  training activity, 157
Bus drivers, 143–144. *See also* Noninstructional personnel

C

Cafeteria workers, 144. *See also* Noninstructional personnel

Catharsis (stage of
    bibliotherapy), 66
Chaos, 24
Children's literature. *See*
    Bibliotherapy
Chronic illness, of students, 79–
    80
Classroom emergency kits, 27
Communication
    barriers to, 45–46
    basic skills, 44–49
    with media, 56–57
    office staff and, 143
    with parents, 55–56, 68
    professional referrals, 45
Concern for students. *See*
    School climate
Conflict resolution, 135, 140
Control, 11, 27
Crisis, defined, 2
Crisis intervention, 1–4, 24,
    147–148, 149
Crisis plans, 24–31. *See also*
    Crisis prevention
Crisis prevention, 3, 4–6, 7–10.
    See also Crisis plans
Crisis teams, 26–27
Cultural diversity. *See* Diver-
    sity concerns
Custodial staff, 144

D

Death, 83–84, 119, 134, 135
Define "Normal" (Peters), 136
Demographics and schools, 32–
    33
Denial, 83–84
Depression, of students, 78
Disabled students, bullying
    and, 7
Diversity concerns
    bibliotherapy and, 66–67,
        135, 136
    crisis intervention and, 31–35
    demographics, 32–33
    identity and, 33–34
    language barriers and, 33
    needs assessment, 34–35
    religion and, 34–35
Divorce, 80–81, 107, 108, 115, 134

E

Emergency kits, 27
Empathy, communication skills
    and, 44–45

F

Faculty training. *See* Training,
    faculty
Fear, 87–88, 131
Financial difficulties, 137, 138,
    139
Flexibility, of crisis plan, 25
Follow-up, communication
    skills and, 48
Friendships, 80, 114, 133

G

Gender concerns, 6–7, 12
Gettin' through Thursday (Coo-
    per), 137
Grieving, 83–84, 119, 120, 127
Guilt, 83–84

H

Handouts
    Bullying, 15
    Decreasing Bullying, 16
    Diversity in Our Schools, 40
    Evaluating Literature for
        Bibliotherapy, 75
    list of, xv–xvi
    Listening to Students in Cri-
        sis: Basic Listening
        Skills, 61
    Preventing Burnout: Keeping
        Yourself Emotionally
        Healthy, 159
    Questions about Your School
        Crisis Plan, 41
    Role Playing Crisis Scenarios,
        42
    Sea Glass, 121
    Topic: Abuse, 116, 117
    Topic: Chronic and Serious
        Illness, 113
    Topic: Death and Grief, 119
    Topic: Depression, 112
    Topic: Difficulties Making
        and Keeping Friends,
        114
    Topic: Divorce, 115
    Topic: Grief, 120
    Topic: Suicide, 118
    Violence, 17
Harassment. *See* Bullying; Sex-
    ual harassment
Hierarchy, crisis planning and,
    26, 27, 28
Home problems, 81

How to Lose All Your Friends
    (Carlson), 133

I

Identification (stage of
    bibliotherapy), 66
Illness, of students, 79–80
Incident Command System
    (ICS), 27
Instability, problems with, 24
Intervention, stages, 3–4
Involvement (stage of
    bibliotherapy), 66
Is It Right to Fight? (Thomas),
    141

J

Joey Pigza Swallowed the Key
    (Gantos), 132

K

Kits, emergency, 27

L

Language barriers. *See* Diver-
    sity concerns
Lilly's Purple Plastic Purse
    (Henkes), 140
Listening skills. *See* Communi-
    cation; Training, faculty
Literature, children's. *See*
    Bibliotherapy

M

Media, communication with,
    56–57
Medications, effects on stu-
    dents, 79–80
Mental health professionals
    referrals, 68
    training, 89–90
Mental illness, 135, 136
Money Hungry (Flake), 138
Multicultural issues. *See* Diver-
    sity concerns
My Louisiana Sky (Holt), 135

N

Nobody Knew What to Do
    (McCain), 22
Noninstructional personnel,
    142–149
Nonverbal communication, 47

R

Ramona and Her Father
    (Cleary), 139
Reactions to stress and trauma.
    See Student response to
    stress and trauma
References, 167–170
Referrals, professional, 68
Reflective listening, communi-
    cation skills and, 45
Religious concerns, 34–35
Resilience, of students, 77–78
Resources. *See also* Activities;
    Handouts; Overheads;
    Worksheets
  avoiding burnout, 158
  bibliotherapy, 72
  communication, 57
  crisis intervention, 161–163
  introduction to crisis inter-
    vention, 13
  noninstructional personnel,
    148–149
  responding to a crisis, 39
  student response to stress
    and trauma, 102–103
Response to crisis
  adults, responsibilities of, 28–29
  crisis plans, 24–25
  crisis teams, 26–27
  diversity concerns, 31–35
  organization, 27
  resources, 39–43
  training, 35–38
Response to stress and trauma.
    See Student response to
    stress and trauma
Responsibilities
  of adults, 28–29
  burnout prevention and, 154–155
Routines, response to stress
    and trauma and, 12

S

Sadness, 83–84
School climate, 4–6. *See also*
    Bullying
School's role in providing men-
    tal health services, vii–ix
Secondary intervention, 3
Self-awareness, burnout pre-
    vention and, 154
Separation. *See* Divorce
Sexual harassment, 7, 20. *See
    also* Bullying

Shame, 83–84
Sincerity, communication skills
    and, 45
Skills inventory of staff, 147
Sleep, stress/trauma and, 11
Speech, communication skills
    and, 48
Staff. *See* Noninstructional per-
    sonnel
Stages, of bibliotherapy, 66
Stigma, 83–84
Stockton schoolyard shootings, 32
Stress. *See* Student response to
    stress and trauma
Stress, employment related, 152
Stress-reducing activities, burn-
    out prevention and, 156
Student response to stress and
    trauma
  abuse, 81–82
  anxiety, 78
  assessing, 26
  bibliotherapy, 68–69, 85
  chronic illness, 79–80
  classroom activities, 86–102
  death and grieving, 83–84
  depression, 78
  divorce and, 80–81
  friendships, 80
  home problems, 81
  medications, 79–80
  reactions, 10–12
  resilience, 77–78
  resources, 102–141
  suicide, 82–83
  table, 11
  training, 84
Suicide, 82–83, 118, 126
Support, burnout prevention
    and, 155–156
Sympathy, communication skills
    and, 44–45

T

Tables, list of, xvii
Teaching techniques,
    bibliotherapy, 67–68
Tertiary intervention, 3–4
Tolerance, bibliotherapy, 134,
    135, 136
Training, faculty
  avoiding burnout, 157
  crisis plan review, 28–29, 35–
    36
  crisis scenario role-play, 36–38
  diversity, 35

Training, faculty *(continued)*
    importance of, 24
    listening skills, 49–54
    specific problems, 84
Training, mental health profes-
    sionals, 89–90
Training, noninstructional per-
    sonnel, 144–146
Trauma. *See* Student response
    to stress and trauma

V

Violence prevention, 17, 21.
    See also Crisis prevention;
    Crisis plans

W

When Addie Was Scared
    (Bailey), 131
*When Zachary Beaver Came to
    Town* (Holt), 134
Worksheets
    Behavior Problems: What,
        Where and How Often,
        14
    Bibliotherapy Summary, 73
    Crisis Intervention: Skills
        Inventory, 149
    Divorce Worksheet (Ages 8–
        12), 107
    Emergency Contact Log, 60

Expressing Our Fee
Feelings about Di
    6–12), 108
list of, xv
Listening Skills
Listening Skill
Masks (Ages
Masks (Ag
Problem-
    8 a
Thoug

We
We